Navigating Nutrition in Later Life

Navigating Nutrition in Later Life

How to stay stronger for longer

Mary Merheim

Navigating Nutrition in Later Life
by Mary Merheim
© Mary Merheim

https://marymerheim.co.uk

Published in 2024 by Mary Merheim

The right of Mary Merheim to be identified as the author of this work has been asserted in accordance with the Copyright, Designs and Patents Act 1988.

All rights reserved. No part of this book may be reproduced, stored in a retrieval system, or transmitted in any form or by any means, electronic, mechanical, photocopying, recording or otherwise, without the prior written permission of the copyright holder.

Book design, typesetting and editing by Jason Conway
www.thedaydreamacademy.com

Contents

Introduction	1
Appetite Loss	7
The Problem with Malnourishment in Old Age	17
Good Nutrition	23
Simple 'Hacks' to Increase Good Nutrition	41
Recipe Suggestions	51
Hydration	75
Helping Someone to Eat	79
Dysphagia in Layman's Terms	85
Final Words	91
Appendix Sample Week Menu	92
Resources and References	93
About the Author	95

Dedication

This book just has to be dedicated to my father, Frederic Arnold Heaton-Merheim (Micky to many friends and family).

My mother died far too young at the age of 58, so he became father and mother to me and my sister, Sarah, aged 21 and 22 at the time. He did this admirably for the next 32 years.

It was an honour and a privilege to support him closely in his final months and to have him try out all my attempts to build him up - when he just didn't fancy eating any more.

Sadly, his heart stopped suddenly and unexpectedly on 10th April 2018, at the age of 90.

Acknowledgements

Thank you to:

- My two daughters: Caty and Emma, who have been chief tasters and put up with me being focussed on looking after the elderly. Much of my time has been spent creating Grandbars® in my father's memory.

- Lisa King 'selfloveologist', Expansion Guide and Mentor who inspired me to write.

- I am deeply grateful to Stirling Gallacher (actor: Doctors, Casualty) for entrusting me with the care of her father during his final months. His struggle with appetite loss inspired me to enhance the nutritional value of small portions, which also contributed to the ongoing development of Grandbar cakes. I also appreciate the entire family, spanning three generations, who generously participated as product testers.

- Jason Conway of The Daydream Academy who has formatted and edited this book and created the cover.

Introduction

There is very little information online about nutrition for anyone over 60 and it can be difficult to know who to ask for advice.

Do you worry about the impact of a low appetite and weight loss on frailty and illness?

I get it…

I gave up teaching in 2016 to look after my father. There wasn't anything particularly wrong with him… he was 88 with a history of bowel and bladder cancer, a bit of COPD and a slight amount of heart failure. He was still doing The Times crossword every day and was fiercely independent. It was just that he'd lost his oomph.

He had been houseproud to the point of obsession, but he had recently told me he couldn't be bothered to make his bed. I can't remember if he was still driving at that point, but, if not then, it wasn't long afterwards that he lost his confidence. He'd had a couple of bumps on a mini roundabout because he thought you took it in turns and I think he'd had a bit of anger towards himself for driving slowly.

Anyway, I think he finally viewed himself as officially old, and with that came feelings of sadness and weariness. The most worrying thing for me was his loss of interest in food. He had been a widower since he was 59 (almost 30 years) and had made himself busy by working as a business consultant, playing golf, and becoming an incredible cook. He was a very curious and scientific chap, and he took his food very seriously. He used to make his own pork pies and beef mince. He'd buy cow's tongues with the tastebuds still on and press them in aspic jelly. He'd also loved his vegetable garden and relished bringing his nurtured creations to the dining table.

By 2017, that love and passion for square meals and savoury dishes had all but vanished. He refused to eat 'ready meals' but didn't want to cook for himself anymore.

I really knew nothing more than the basics about nutrition at that time… least of all in the elderly. All I knew was that I was watching him fade away in front of me, for no good reason that I could see. I knew he was nearly 90 but it still seemed his decline in weight and subsequent health could be turned around, if only I knew how. Millionaire's Shortbread was the one thing that he actually looked forward to eating. I didn't mind buying it for him as, at least, his calorie intake was going up. However, nutritional value was zero!

After a little while, I searched on the internet for granola bar, energy ball and tray bake recipes that I could adapt, to tempt and nourish him. I got tinkering in the kitchen and involved him in the bashing, grinding, and mixing of enormous amounts of ingredients over the next few months. We tried, tasted, and modified our creations with teamwork and hilarity. He grew stronger and his interest in things culinary returned somewhat.

While looking up the recipes, I also researched nutrition in the elderly and discovered this is a hugely neglected topic, with sparse real studies or easily accessible information. Even the NHS website lacked guidelines for calories, vitamins and nutrients for the 'over 60's'.

Although I reignited my father's interest in some foods, had a blast with him and stopped his weight loss, I couldn't prevent the inevitable. In April 2018 he suffered a sudden and unexpected heart attack, at the age of 90. Thankfully, I was with him and can only describe it as a Good Death, especially as he had completed his beloved Times crossword a couple of hours earlier!

As a result of this, I retrained as a carer and became a self-employed Dementia and End of Life Doula. Supporting families in this way is an absolute pleasure and a privilege, and something I still do. However, my passion for learning about the nutrition of the elderly just grew and grew. I knew, from personal experience, the significance and detrimental effects of a low appetite and not eating well in later years, and wanted to help others. I had researched, and seen, how and why people lose their appetite and how it affects not just the older generation but the people who care for them too.

I've also learnt that our systems need to be nourished in slightly different ways as we age. More protein and more of most nutrients, with only a slight dip in calorie requirements. The quality of every mouthful needs to be considered, as we are less able to extract and absorb the 'good stuff' from our food. Every mouthful matters.

I continued my development of the cake bars I'd started making with my father, and in June 2022, thanks (in a not unsubstantial part) to his legacy, I started selling Grandbars® online and at food festivals. They immediately earned the runner up spot for a 'healthy boost' product at the Great British Food Awards, and won Start Up of the Year at the 2023 Gloucestershire Foodie

Awards. I now have a very experienced management team and the business is growing.

In October 2023, I passed my HND (level 5) in Nutrition and became a Nutrition Advisor to the Elderly. I give professional development talks to staff in care agencies and care homes, fun and informative talks to voluntary organisations and social groups, including the Women's Institute, as well as personal one-to-one guidance.

Appetite Loss

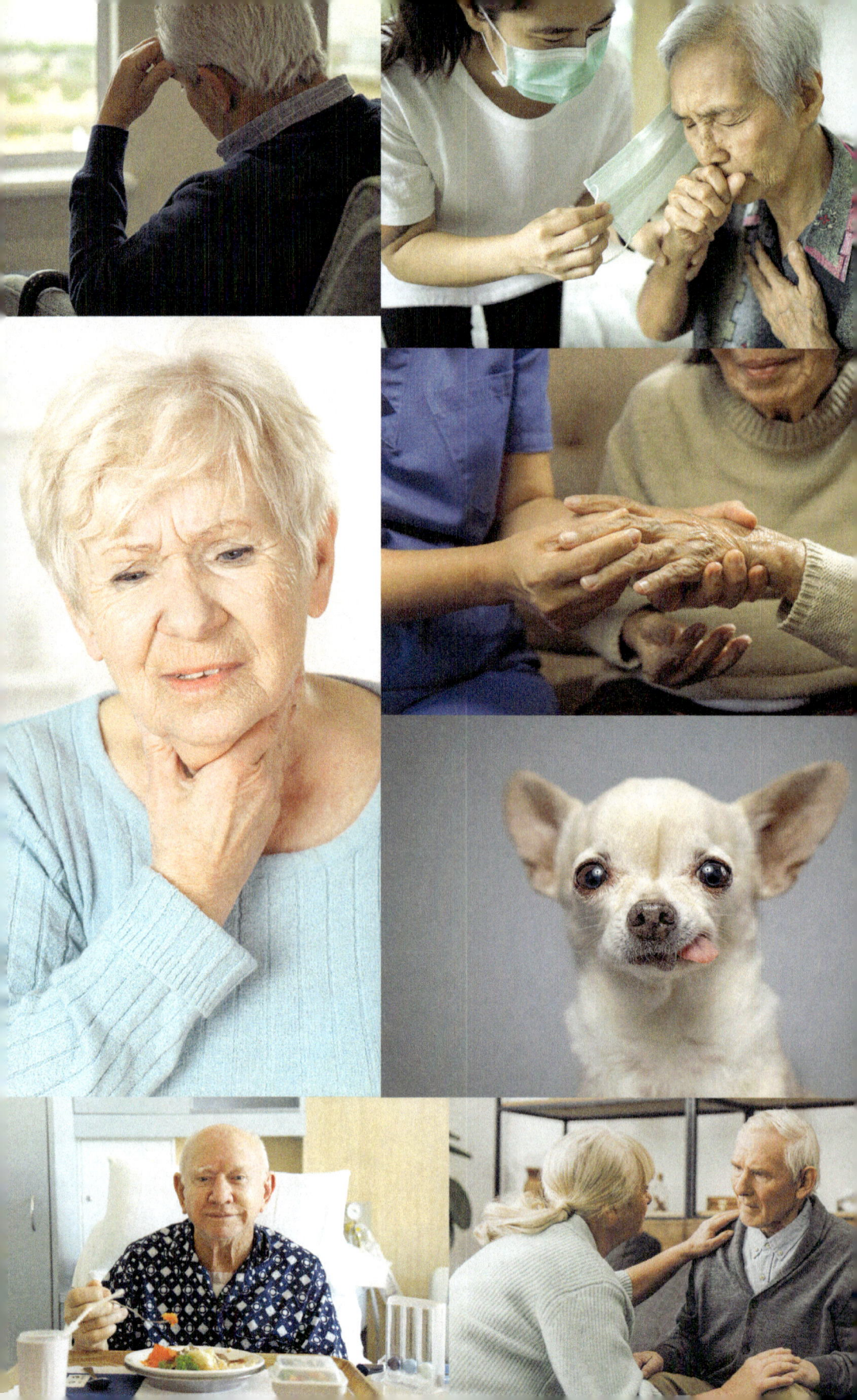

Appetite Loss

Myth: Loss of appetite is normal as we get older. It is usually thought that less activity will naturally cause appetite loss and is not a concern.

Absolutely not. Loss of appetite is down to many complex issues.

Although it is not 'normal', it is, indeed, extremely common.

Quite often, it doesn't get noticed until things start to go awry, so it is useful to keep an eye on common signs of thinness:

- bones visible under the skin
- clothes becoming baggy and ill-fitting
- needing a belt for trousers when they didn't before, making new holes in older belts
- rings and dentures becoming loose

Appetite can go down in later years for so many reasons and some are easier to 'fix' than others.

1. Loneliness and depression.
It can be very hard living alone. Self care can slip when it becomes harder work and there's no one else affected by it. The older generation were very much part of a more traditional way of life. Even right up to the 1980's, women tended to do the cooking and care for their husbands, while the men went out to work. If a man lost his wife, he may simply not know how to make healthy and varied meals. Conversely, a woman may feel she has no one to cook for. When your life has had order for many years,

and this is taken away from you, it is difficult to adapt and change.

Sadness, loneliness and grief all affect your emotions and your body. You may simply not feel hungry, as well as feeling disinclined to care for yourself properly.

Obviously, the fix here is multifaceted and complicated. Eating a meal, historically, is a social activity and not just for sustenance. If you are visiting a relative, always plan to take a meal to share or at least tea and cake! It has been proven that we eat more in company than alone, so maybe think about suggesting a lunch club or day centre.

2. Medication.
Many medications can have side effects that include suppressing your appetite. These include:

- Antibiotics
- Chemotherapy
- Digoxin, given to control irregular heartbeats
- Fluoxetine, an antidepressant
- Hydralazine, for high blood pressure and heart issues
- Opioids and other strong painkillers
- Metformin and other drugs for Type 2 Diabetes

Have a chat with the GP and have all medication reviewed. Sometimes just a change of brand, or tweaking the dose, may reduce the side effects.

3. Short term and long term health conditions.
Short term illnesses and injuries can stop us wanting to eat.

Infections like flu, common colds, urine infections, chest infections, and tummy bugs can all have dramatic effects on appetite. Short term issues like sore throats and headaches can also mean you don't want to eat.

When I was young, the 'cure all' was Lucozade! Ensure you are drinking lots of fluids, preferably with electrolytes. If loss of appetite from an acute illness is an issue for more than a few days, then you will need to seek medical advice.

Lots of long term conditions also have a huge impact on how much and what you eat. I'm listing the more common ones linked to aging, as opposed to lifelong ones like Crohn's Disease or Coeliac Disease.

- Conditions causing breathlessness. If it is hard to breathe, it is hard to eat at the same time as breathe. If it is difficult to breathe, it may be hard to eat at the same time as breathe. Medicalconditions causing this might include chronic obstructive pulmonary disease (COPD), pneumonia, asthma, pulmonary embolism, and congestive heart failure.

- Acid reflux and indigestion. This becomes very common as we get older. Gallstones can also cause severe pain, particularly after eating fatty foods.

- Cancer. Many different cancers can cause a loss of appetite. Usually, a low appetite is accompanied by other symptoms specific to the location of the tumour, but sometimes not wanting to eat can be an early symptom of cancer too.

- Constipation. As we get older, our stomach is more slow to empty. Our whole digestive system slows down and becomes less efficient. Constipation can have other, and wider, effects, such as mood changes, pain and sickness.

- Liver disease. The early symptoms of liver disease include feeling sick (nausea), feeling tired, diarrhoea, as well as appetite loss.

For all short and long term issues, the best approach is gentle but highly nutritious food – little and often.

4. Chewing Problems (Dysphagia).

Any problems that make it difficult to swallow might interfere with appetite. For example, just in the mouth, there might be problems with toothache, poorly fitting dentures, dental abscesses, a dry mouth or weak jaw.

All these issues are best checked out by a dentist, however, mobility problems may make visiting the dentist harder than ever. The older person may worry about the expense too. Simple, short term tricks that might ease the pain are swilling the mouth with salty water and using over the counter numbing gels, but these really are temporary measures. Dry mouth is a very common problem and you can easily buy great saliva replacement gels, or sweets, from a pharmacist or online. Choose food that requires little chewing.

It is a very good idea to ask to be referred to a Speech and Language Therapist (SaLT) through the GP / Community Nurse / Frailty Team. They will have ideas and equipment /

utensils to help with the physical side of chewing, swallowing and drinking. There, the International Dysphagia Diet Standardisation Initiative (IDDSI) offers guidelines and support with eating softer food.

5. Taste Changes.

Changes in how you actually taste things are extremely common. As we age, our tastebuds deteriorate (along with the rest of the body) with the savoury receptors weakening first. This means that food you once might have loved like meat, cheeses, breads and vegetables, can start to taste quite bland or even unpleasant.

Add more flavours, herbs and spices to foods. Try adding honey or fruit to traditionally savoury dishes.

6. Lack of physical strength.

Not eating well, snacking and not cooking for oneself may simply be because someone has lost strength or feeling in their fingers, wrists or arms. Picking up a saucepan, or frying pan, might just feel too dangerous to anyone with issues in this area. Even picking up a hot plastic contained ready meal from the microwave might be too much of a strain.

I have been round to many clients' homes and the bottom line is they can't open a tin any more because the opener needs one hand to squeeze it, and the other to turn it! I have to go into some people's fridges to open their milk bottles and packets of cheese and ham for them. Think how difficult it is to rip those tiny sachets of ketchup and mayonnaise. That is how a lot of packaging feels to older hands.

There is a wonderful world out there of gadgets and aids to help with this. Wide and soft handled cutlery; easy-use cups, mugs and plates, as well as implements you might never have thought of. A quick internet search will find so many things to make the kitchen an easier and safer place.

7. Being somewhere different.

It is a very common problem that older people struggle when they first arrive in hospital, or in a supported living situation. However good it might be, institutional food is just not the same as being at home. With the best will in the world, meals will be served up at different times, in different ways, from what you are used to (I am being very careful not to go down the rabbit hole of discussing the quality of hospital / care home food, or the expertise / time / budgets that the staff may have. That is a book in itself!). There are distractions, noises and routines that can be really unsettling, as well as unfamiliar faces and voices.

It depends on personality really! For some people, you might want to ensure there are reasonably healthy snacks available at all times. For others, it might be better if they 'tough it out' and adapt more quickly to new routines. As with all things, a sensible compromise of the two will be best in most cases. Obviously, it also depend on the quality of taste, texture, look, and nutritional content of the food being served. Also, see if there is a way of easing gently into the new routine: somewhere quiet to sit, having your familiar place setting, some meals in your room, or a meal 'buddy' (either a member of staff or someone of a similar age).

8. Dementia.

This is a really common cause of not eating / not eating healthily.

Dementia UK has published the following list of reasons people may not eat well with dementia:

They might....

- forget to eat or drink
- not recognise when they are hungry, thirsty or full
- have trouble preparing food or drinks
- struggle to recognise food items
- find certain colours, textures or smells of food off-putting
- struggle to follow particular diets, for example, for diabetes, coeliac disease, or religious / cultural diets
- have difficulty handling cutlery and feeding themselves
- find it difficult to swallow
- develop a sweet tooth

Dementia UK also suggest the following ways you can help:

You could try:

- *involving the person in deciding what to eat – you could suggest two options:*
    - *getting them to help prepare food*
    - *offering a small snack before a meal. This may help them realise they're hungry*
- *providing foods with different tastes, smells and colours to stimulate their appetite*
- *giving them small, regular portions, rather than large meals*
- *turning off the TV to avoid distractions*
- *playing some soothing, familiar music*
- *planning mealtimes to avoid times when the person*

- *may be tired or distressed*
- *allowing plenty of time to eat*
- *eating with the person – but bear in mind some people may be self-conscious about eating in company*
- *making sure the room is well-lit*
- *using plain coloured plates so they can see the food easily (red is often good)*
- *giving them finger food*
- *trying adapted cutlery for people with dementia*

The Problem with Malnourishment in Old Age

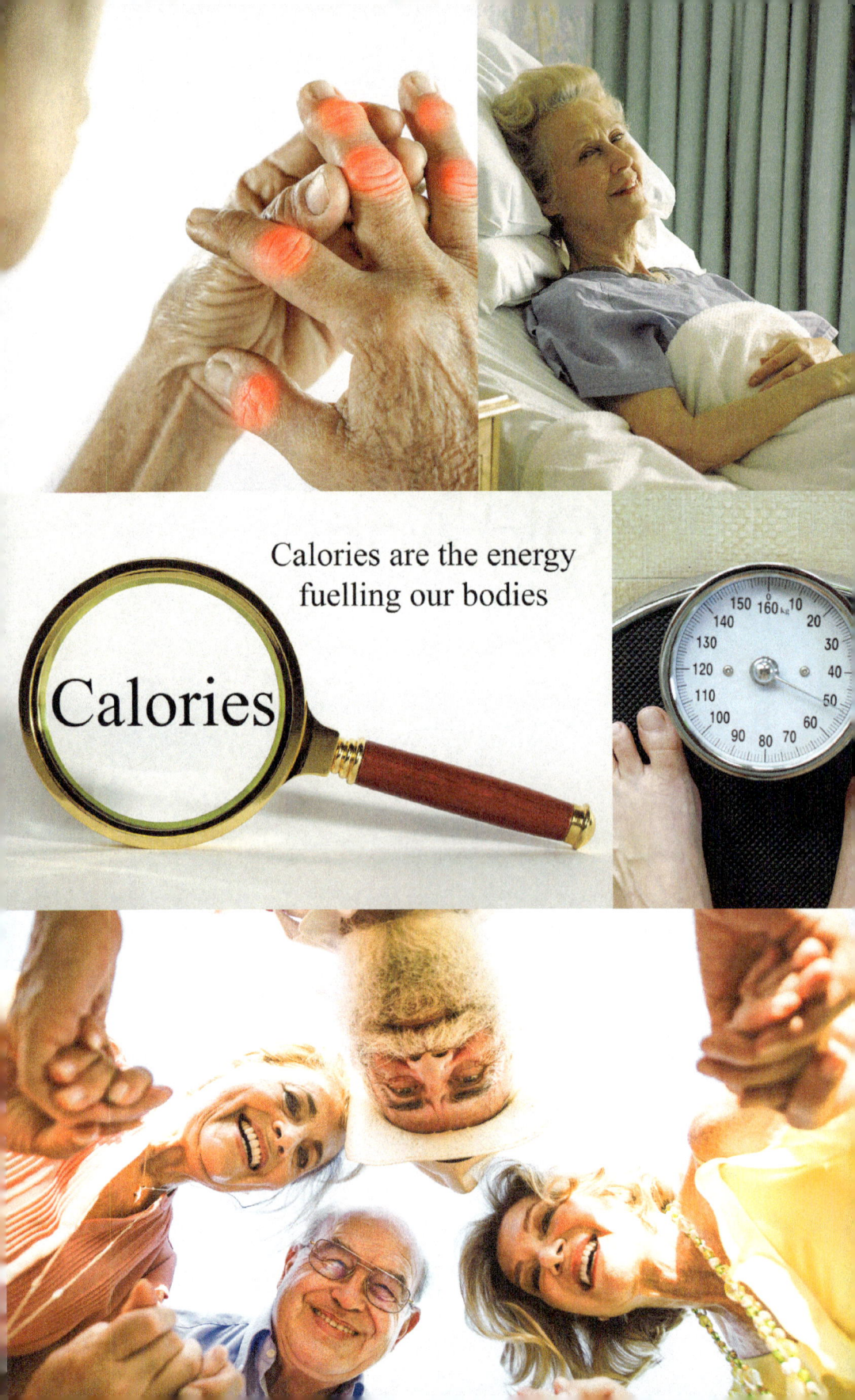

The Problem with Malnourishment in Old Age

Myth: Slower metabolism means you need fewer calories.

Wrong! Calorific needs are, actually, only slightly decreased. In fact, due to the digestive system becoming less efficient, highly nutrient dense food becomes more important. Good quality regular food is vital in later years.

Old Age.
First off... what is old age? When is it? The World Health Organisation (WHO) initially attempted to come up with an internationally agreed definition. The best they could do was that "old age" is denoted by the age of 60–65 years in the developed world". Other studies have further subdivided into:

Young Old: 60-69 years

Middle Old: 70-79 years

Very Old 80+ years

As our bodies age, although the calorie requirement may go very slightly down (as you will see later), the nutrient requirement goes up. Not only do our minds and bodies need more help to slow down the aging processes and fight off infection, our gut gets less efficient at absorbing nutrients.

The World Health Organisation defines malnutrition as: deficiencies, excesses or imbalances in a person's intake of energy and / or nutrients.

According to the British Association for Parenteral and Enteral Nutrition (BAPEN), and the Malnutrition Task Force, 1 in 10 people over 65 in the UK are currently affected by malnutrition.

Symptoms of Malnutrition.
Symptoms of poor nutrition are not just weight loss. Eating sausage and mash all day, every day, might stop you looking underweight, and you may even have a reasonable BMI, but you would still be malnourished. In fact, symptoms of poor nutrition can be very subtle and be seen as just signs of getting older.

Particular signs of poor nutrition can be:

- Weight loss. An obvious one, but it's not always the case
- Dry skin and hair
- Brittle / soft nails
- Irritability and depression
- Worsening night vision
- Joint pain
- Sores around the mouth

Impact of Poor Nutrition.
If older people do not eat enough, they become under-nourished. This can lead to:

- an increased risk of infection
- poor or slow wound-healing – particularly of ulcers and bedsores
- slow recovery after operations
- skin problems and sores
- breathing difficulties
- muscle weakness, making tasks of daily living more

difficult
- tiredness, confusion and irritability

Poor nutrition has a massive effect on morbidity, regardless of BMI. Malnutrition is associated with longer hospital stays and readmissions. It is responsible for high demands on medical services and early entry to care homes. Chronic disability, frailty, pain, and poor quality of life, are serious consequences of malnutrition, particularly undernutrition. It has also emerged as a significant factor in the development of sarcoma (cancer that starts in the bone or connective tissue) and dementia.

As you can see, we might just attribute most of these symptoms / effects to 'old age'. As we get older, we do, of course, face a variety of health challenges. Blood pressure naturally rises and the immune system becomes weaker, so we may have more difficulty battling invaders and infections. The skin becomes thinner and more wrinkled and may take longer to heal after injury. Older adults may gradually lose an inch or two in height. Short-term memory is often not as sharp as it once was. All these signs of aging are also exacerbated by a lack of nutrients and the reason why good nutrition is so important.

Calorific Requirements.
According to many sources of medical advice, the average man (of average age) should consume 2500 calories a day, and a woman 2000.

Surprisingly, this doesn't change a huge amount as we age. According to the NHS, moderately active men between 46 and 65 years require approximately 2,400 calories each day. After 65, the calorie requirement reduces to about 2,200 calories per day.

For women, the advice seems to be to drop calorie intake to 1800 in their 50's and maintain this through the years.

Obviously, if you become 'bedbound' and totally inactive, the calorific needs of the body drop off. A research paper published in *The Journals of Gerontology* studied the calorific requirements of immobile elderly patients, and found we need 750 kcal just to maintain basic bodily functions.

However, as soon as you have a bed sore, or an injury, calorie requirements go shooting back up to anything from 1000 to 2500, depending on person's weight and type of injury. If you have a fever, you need more calories to make up for your higher body temperature. Even fighting off the common cold takes energy.

In other words... as we age beyond our 50's, our calorific requirements actually decline very slowly. Then, even just lying in bed and immobile, we still need minimum of 750 calories a day for our bodies to do just the very basic tasks of living. However, in order to fight sores, infection, illness, and injury, we need to eat many more calories than the basic requirement.

Good Nutrition

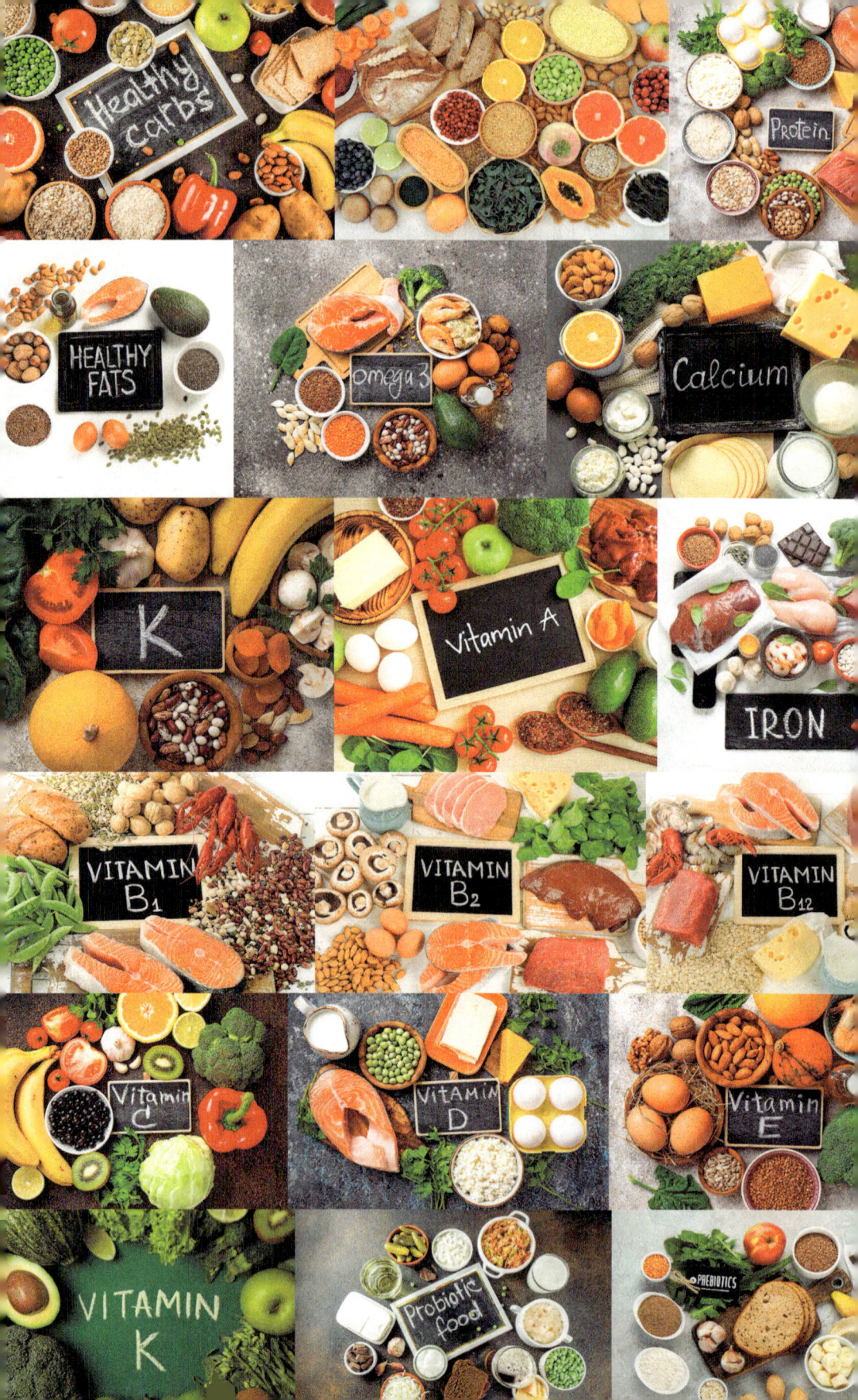

Good Nutrition

Myth: Nutrition can't have that big an impact on the ageing process and dying.

Oh it does. Malnutrition plays a major part in negative prognosis in illness and injury. It is associated with longer hospital stays, re-admission, immune dysfunction, high demands on medical services, and early institutionalization.

As with all scientific theories, research will always be found somewhere that proves or disproves them. I have read a variety of papers published by reliable medical sources and am using them to explain to you, as best I can, what I have learned about the impact of different nutrients.

1. Carbohydrates/Fibre.
Carbohydrates are our main source of energy. There are simple carbohydrates and complex carbohydrates.

- Simple carbohydrates are short chain sugars that are easy to digest and broken down into energy quickly. They can be found naturally in soft fruit, honey, and milk, or created into processed sugar. They do tend to cause spikes and dips in blood sugar levels but aren't all bad.

- Complex Carbohydrates are made up of longer sugar chains (also called starch), so take longer to digest, thus, releasing the sugars / energy more slowly. They can be found naturally in rice and other grains, bread, pasta, starchy and green vegetables, and fruit like bananas and apples.

We are told to eat whole grain complex carbohydrates in order to maximise our nutrition. Unfortunately, eating healthily, particularly in later years, is not simply about replacing simple carbohydrates with complex ones. Natural sources of simple carbohydrates also tend to have nutrients and gentle fibres that are essential. Conversely, some sources of complex carbohydrates have a very low nutritional value, for example: chips, crisps, white rice and white bread.

Older adults are recommended to consume between 45% and 65% of their daily calories as complex carbohydrates. However, if you do have a low appetite, it is best to cut down on bulky carbohydrates like bread and turn to foods that provide carbohydrate, along with protein, fats and nutrients. This could be pulses, legumes, nuts and cheese.

Not eating enough carbohydrates will make you feel shaky, weak and dizzy. You might also feel anxious and hungry. Too much carbohydrate in your diet will lead to craving fatty food, depression and weakening of the muscles.

- Fibre. Complex carbohydrates are 'complex', not just because the sugar molecules are long, but because they contain material the body can't digest, which is fibre. Fibre bulks and softens the stools, preventing constipation. Constipation can be a real problem as we age. In order to add fibre to your diet, it is best to eat leafy greens, fruit and oats. Wholegrain wheat is not particularly suitable when the digestive system weakens. It is very rough and can even cause abrasions and tears in some cases. Oats are much better. They contain higher levels of dietary fibre, protein, minerals, and antioxidants, making them a more nutritious choice.

Great sources of carbohydrates and fibre are oats, lentils, chickpeas, peas, sweet potatoes and butternut squash. When it comes to fruit, some of the best are blueberries, bananas, strawberries and apples. Although most fruit and vegetables are better eaten raw, it has been shown that cooking (stewing apples) releases pectin which can actually help repair and maintain the intestinal mucosa lining and gut microbiomes.

2. Protein.

Protein is the most important nutrient in later years. It is an important part of a healthy diet. Proteins are made up of chemical 'building blocks' called amino acids. Your body uses these amino acids to build and repair skin, muscles and bones, and to make hormones. Without enough, the skin becomes more fragile, immunity function is decreased, wounds and injuries don't heal and it takes longer to recover from illness. Body muscle mass also decreases in later years, so the risk of frailty and falls goes up.

An American study, published in 2017, followed nearly 2,000 older adults over six years. It found that people who consumed the least amount of protein were almost twice as likely to have difficulty walking or climbing steps as those who ate the most (after adjusting for health behaviours, chronic conditions and other factors).[1] The University of Sheffield produced a later study in February 2020 that found that "more than half of older people don't consume enough protein to stay healthy" [2].

Because of the reasons above, research suggests increasing the recommended intake of protein by up to 50 percent in later years. That means people over age 65 should aim for 0.45 to

0.55 gram of protein per pound of body weight daily, or about 68 to 83 grams for a 150-pound person. It is recommended that during illness, and when recovering from injuries such as fractures or skin abrasions (including ulcers, bed sores and other open wounds), the amount of protein should be raised even more.

Beef, chicken, fish and seafood, eggs, dairy, soya, nuts and seeds are great sources of protein.

3. Fats.

Fat is an essential part of a healthy, balanced diet. Fat is a source of essential fatty acids, some of which the body cannot make itself. Fat helps the body absorb vitamin A, vitamin D and vitamin E. These vitamins are fat-soluble, which means they can only be absorbed with the help of fats. Fat also helps give your body energy, protects your organs, supports cell growth, and keeps cholesterol and blood pressure under control. It is particularly important for brain function.

We fear fat because we know all the dangers of being overweight, the risk of heart disease and the word cholesterol. However, there are three types of fat... saturated fat, monounsaturated fat and polyunsaturated fat, as well as two main types of cholesterol.

- LDL (low-density lipoprotein) cholesterol, sometimes called "bad" cholesterol, makes up most of your body's cholesterol. It is a soft, waxy substance that can cause clogged, or blocked, arteries (blood vessels).

- HDL (high-density lipoprotein) cholesterol, sometimes

called "good" cholesterol, absorbs LDL cholesterol in the blood and carries it back to the liver to be broken down and eliminated.

a. Saturated Fat.

Saturated fat tends to be hard and builds up your 'bad' cholesterol. It comes from fatty meat, sausages and bacon as well as in processed foods like cakes, biscuits and pastries.

b. Monounsaturated Fat / Omega-9 Fatty Acids.

Monounsaturated fat can help lower your LDL (bad) cholesterol level. Keeping your LDL level low reduces your risk of heart disease and stroke. Monounsaturated fats help develop and maintain your cells. The body can make its own Omega-9, but it is beneficial to get it from foods as well.

The best everyday sources of Omega-9 fats are nuts, seeds, avocados and olive oil.

c. Polyunsaturated Fat / Omega-3, Omega-6 Fatty Acids.

Omega-3 and Omega-6 fatty acids are polyunsaturated fats associated with several health benefits. Omega-3 fats are essential fats that have important benefits for your heart, brain, and metabolism. Omega-3 dilates (widens) blood vessels and thins the blood. Omega-6 constricts blood vessels and aids with clotting. Both are vital. Both need to be eaten to keep us healthier. While Omega-6 fats provide your body with energy, they are also abundant in our diet. Whereas, most people don't consume enough Omega-3.

Polyunsaturated fats are best known for their role in maintaining heart health by removing built up waste from blood vessels and lowering blood pressure. One of the other key benefits of Omega-3 is helping to keep our body's cell membranes pliable, so the white blood cells can easily pass through blood vessels to fight inflammation [3]. Omega-3 can also keep skin supple and hydrated, aiding the prevention and healing of any sort of wounds [4].

Omega-3 helps the body produce melatonin – the sleep hormone [5]. People with low Omega-3 have been shown to have a higher chance of sleep apnea [6].

Also, although more research is needed, some studies have proved that omega-3 can help with brain function and slow memory loss. It is thought that increasing Omega-3 on diagnosis of Alzheimers Disease can help slow its progress. It supports the way nerves communicate with each other in the brain and low levels of Omega-3 have been found in people with Alzheimers Disease [7,8].

Omega-6 fatty acids can be found in sunflower oil, sunflower seeds, walnuts, eggs, pumpkin seeds, peanut butter and tofu.

Omega-3 fatty acids can be found in Oily fish such as salmon, herring, mackerel, sardines; fish oil, eggs, walnuts, spinach and chia seeds, among other sources. However, the richest source of Omega-3 in the world is flaxseed. Omega-3 supplements are readily available, but can have some side effects like stomach cramps. For optimal Omega-3 fatty acids, it is best to eat 2 portions of oily fish a week, plus regular helpings of walnuts, spinach, eggs and flaxseeds.

5. Calcium.

We all know that calcium is good for bones and teeth, but it can also contribute to the health of the skin, blood and brain. However, increasing intake significantly as we get older is a highly contentious issue. There was a study completed in 2015 that showed increasing calcium in later life did not necessarily improve bone density or risk of fracture. Having said that, it is still important to consume calcium rich food throughout life. The underlying message was that the calcium is needed earlier in life to have an impact on bone health in later years [9].

Women's bone density is particularly at risk during menopause, so during perimenopause and menopause is a great time to look at increasing calcium consumption to help prevent osteoporosis.

Calcium supplements are not always a safe way to add this mineral to your diet. Too much calcium can cause nausea, stomach cramps and kidney stones. There are a few studies that suggest supplements might increase women's risk of heart failure, but these have not been repeated enough to prove the findings.

Dairy is, without a doubt, a very natural and easy way to ensure good levels of calcium. One average glass provides a third of most people's calcium for the day. Green vegetables and seeds are also high in calcium.

6. Iron.

Iron is a vital nutrient for the body, as it is needed to make the red blood cells that carry oxygen around the body. A low level of iron in the body results in anaemia. Anaemia is extremely common in older people. This is a huge health worry as it can cause light headedness, falls, rapid heart rate, shortness of breath, headaches and chest pain.

There are lots of reasons why you might get anaemic in later life:

- Eating less iron rich food. Red meat and liver are very high in iron but, as I've mentioned before, savoury tastebuds deteriorating may make meat taste unpleasantly metallic. Red meat usually needs chewing which can be difficult as we age, plus we are advised to eat less red meat because of its cholesterol content.

- Bleeding. Not only does skin become thinner and bruises / bleeds more easily, but many older people are on blood thinners that mean you bleed even more heavily. Also, the digestive tract becomes thinner and ulcers become more likely, leading to a certain amount of internal bleeding. Some medications, or combinations of medications, can increase the risk of internal bleeding too. Ibuprofen, paracetamol and aspirin are common drugs that can lead to internal bleeding, but others linked to it are antibiotics, antidepressants, statins and acid reflux meds (proton pump inhibitors like Omeprazole).

- Any sort of disease or infection, be it chronic or short term, affects our absorption of vital nutrients.

Iron is found in all meats, leafy vegetables and legumes (beans, peas and lentils). Dried fruits, such as prunes, raisins, and apricots are also great sources of iron.

5. Potassium.

Potassium is a positively charged electrolyte. Electrolytes are minerals that have a negative or positive charge when dissolved in water, or other body fluids, such as blood. It helps carry an electric charge through your body. It helps:

- Muscles expand and contract
- Move nutrients into, and waste out of, your cells
- Reverse the effect of salt (sodium) on your blood pressure
- Nerves send messages from the brain to the body, and back again

Potassium is a strange one as older people can be prone to too low, or too high, levels.

Low potassium is usually caused by taking diuretics for high blood pressure. In this instance, studies have shown that taking potassium supplements don't help, as the diuretics will still eliminate them and other electrolytes [10]. Potassium will be low in anyone not eating or drinking optimally. Vomiting can also trigger potassium loss from urine, which makes prolonged vomiting result in low potassium levels.

Potassium deficiency symptoms usually develop slowly in the elderly with signs such as fatigue, muscle weakness, cramps, bone fragility, nausea, vomiting, and higher blood sugar. Low potassium can also cause several mood changes in older adults, including confusion, depression, nervous disorders, and erratic behaviour.

To increase potassium, eat a high-potassium diet, which includes foods such as avocados, melons, bananas, broccoli,

spinach, granola, kidney beans, milk, nuts, oranges, peanut butter, potatoes, pumpkin, raisins, tomatoes and tuna.

High potassium (Hyperkalymia) is usually caused by decreased kidney function. As you age, your kidneys may lose their ability to filter blood, and may have problems with excreting potassium. Some medications like non-steroidal anti-inflammatory drugs can increase potassium too. It can also be a result of eating too high a potassium diet, such as large amounts of tomatoes, bananas, yogurt, citrus fruit and meats. These can cause too much potassium to enter your blood. Salt substitutes are also high in potassium and can cause issues for individuals who cannot adequately excrete potassium.

Other (less common) causes include:

- Taking extra potassium, such as salt substitutes or supplements.

- A disorder called "Addisons disease", which affects your adrenal glands.

- Burns or other severe injuries. This occurs because your body, in response to severe burns or injuries, releases extra potassium in your blood to aid healing.

- Poorly controlled diabetes.

- When diabetes is not controlled, it has a direct effect on your kidneys which are responsible for balancing potassium and sodium in your body.

High Potassium often has no specific symptoms, other than feeling tired, weaker, slightly sick or numbness / tingling in the body. If hyperkalemia comes on suddenly, and you have very high levels of potassium, you may feel heart palpitations, shortness of breath, chest pain, nausea or vomiting. Sudden or severe hyperkalemia is a life-threatening condition. It requires immediate medical care.

The presence of high potassium is usually discovered by chance, through a routine blood check.

To lower your potassium reduce / avoid dairy, chocolate, nuts, seeds and the other high potassium foods mentioned above. Drinking tea, coffee and sparkling water helps too.

6. Vitamin A / Retinol / Beta-Carotene.

Vitamin A is vital for your immune system and keeping your skin and mucous membranes healthy. It also helps vision in dim light.

If you consume a lot of vitamin A, your body can store it, so it is not so important to eat vitamin A rich food every day. In rare instances of having too much, it can lead to bone weakness.

Mild deficiency in Vitamin A can cause fatigue and susceptibility to infection. More severe deficiency can lead to dry eyes, poor night vision and dry skin.

Retinols are an easy-to-absorb form of Vitamin A. They are found in dairy, eggs and oily fish, as well as some fortified cereals. The myth that was created about carrots being good for your eyesight is actually true, as they are a great source of carotenoids that can be converted by the body to make

Vitamin A. Other sources are red fruits (including tomatoes), broccoli and sweet potatoes.

7. Vitamin Bs and B12.

The main B vitamins are also known as Thiamin, Riboflavin, Niacin and Folate, as well as Vitamin B12.

- Thiamin or Vitamin B1 helps the body release energy from food and keeps the nervous system healthy.

Good sources are peas, nuts and liver.

- Riboflavin, or Vitamin B2, does the same as thiamin, plus is good for skin and eyes.

Good sources are milk, eggs, mushrooms and yoghurt. UV light can destroy riboflavin, so these foods should be kept out of sunlight.

- Niacin or Vitamin B3 is needed for the same things as Riboflavin.

It can be found in meat, fish, wheat and eggs.

- Folate, or Vitamin B9, helps the body form healthy red blood cells. A lack can lead to folate deficiency anaemia, which is the same as for a B12 deficiency. Manmade folate (Folic Acid) is often given to pregnant women.

Folate is in all leafy green vegetables, chickpeas, kidney beans and liver. All of these B vitamins are usually added to 'fortified cereal'.

- Vitamin B12 is also needed for creating red blood cells and DNA. Low levels can cause (or be a result of) pernicious anaemia.

As we get older, our ability to absorb vitamin B12 decreases. This is because aging adults often develop problems with the acids and stomach enzymes needed to process the vitamin. All heartburn medicines, including proton pump inhibitors (PPIs), decrease the stomach's ability to absorb B12. We can store B12 in our liver for up to 5 years but a poorly functioning liver, due to alcohol intake, age or disease, can have a detrimental impact on this.

Mild Vitamin B12 deficiency may show no symptoms. If untreated, you can go on to develop:

- Tiredness, weakness or lightheadedness
- Pale skin
- Heart palpitations and shortness of breath
- Loss of appetite, constipation or diarrhoea
- Muscle weakness, numbness or tingling
- Very smooth tongue and mouth ulcers
- Vision problems
- Memory loss, depression or changes in behaviour

Often solutions are injections of B12 by the GP, or high dose edible supplements. Prevention can be boosted by eating meats, dairy, eggs and seafood. If you don't eat these things, another source is fortified breakfast cereal.

8. Vitamin C.
Vitamin C is an antioxidant that helps protect your cells against

the effects of free radicals. Free radicals are unstable molecules produced naturally when your body breaks down foods. However, they are also created by cigarette smoke, radiation (including from the sun) and pollutants which are all easily absorbed by the body. They can play a role in heart disease, cancer, and other diseases if not broken down and eliminated. Vitamin C also helps your body absorb and store iron. Also called Ascorbic Acid, it helps maintain healthy bones, cartilage, skin and blood vessels.

The problem is that our bodies can't store Vitamin C, as it can with most other vitamins and minerals. We have to consume it every day to keep our levels high enough. This means eating fresh or frozen fruit and vegetables.

A UK government survey, in the late 1990's, of people aged over 65 found that 4% – that was almost half a million – had vitamin C deficiency, which is technically defined as below 11 mcmol/l. That figure rose significantly in residential care homes, where an estimated 40% were found to have vitamin C levels below 11 µmol/l [11].

A survey conducted recently in the USA, in 2023, found pretty much the same results. Older 'institutionalised' people were found to have quite significant deficiencies [12].

Citrus fruits contain high amounts of vitamin C but can also cause diarrhoea in large amounts. Other sources include leafy vegetables, potatoes and peppers. In this instance, vitamin C supplements are a way in which people can healthily add it to their diet.

9. Vitamin D.

Calcium can only be absorbed if the body has sufficient amounts of vitamin D. Vitamin D is a fat soluble vitamin that aids calcium uptake. With low vitamin D, the body can only absorb 10-15% of calcium from food sources, whereas, with vitamin D, that improves to 30-40%. Generally, we get much of our vitamin D from sunlight. As we become more housebound, and less inclined to spend any length of time outdoors, we need to increase our level of edible vitamin D.

To add vitamin D to the diet, to help the absorption of calcium, this can be found in oily fish, red meat, liver, eggs, oranges and bananas. Current UK Government advice is that anyone who is not often outdoors (frail or housebound), in a hospital or care home, should take a daily Vitamin D supplement.

10. Vitamin E.

Vitamin E helps maintain healthy skin and eyes, and strengthens the immune system. It is a fat soluble antioxidant that helps the body deal with free radicals (see Vitamin C). There have also been studies to suggest supplements can help reduce Non Alcoholic Fatty Liver Disease (NAFLD) [13].

However, high doses of Vitamin E may have negative interactions with anticoagulant / antiplatelet medications; simvastatin and cancer treatments. There is also some study to suggest it may increase the risk of prostate cancer [14].

Natural sources of Vitamin E are all plant oils, nuts and seeds, and wheatgerm.

11. Vitamin K.

Vitamin K is a fat soluble vitamin that is needed in blood clotting and helping wounds to heal. It can be stored in the liver for later use, so need not be ingested every day.

It is found in leafy greens, vegetable oils and cereal.

12. Probiotics and Prebiotics.

Prebiotics stimulate and feed the microbiomes to make them healthy and reproduce.

According to the NHS, there is very little evidence that eating probiotics actually changes the gut flora in most people. However some studies show they might help Irritable Bowel Disease (IBD) and diarrhoea caused by antibiotics.

Probiotics are added to many live yoghurts. They are also found in fermented food such as kimchi, kifir and sauerkraut.

Here are some of the most common prebiotics and where you can find them:

- *Fructooligosaccharides (FOS) – asparagus, onions, leeks, garlic, bananas, Jerusalem artichokes, chicory root*
- *Galactooligossaccharides (GOS) – legumes like chickpeas and lentils*
- *Inulin – asparagus, onions, leeks, garlic, bananas, Jerusalem artichokes, chicory root*
- *Beta-glucan – some mushrooms, barley, oats, rye, and other whole grains*

Simple 'Hacks' to Increase Good Nutrition

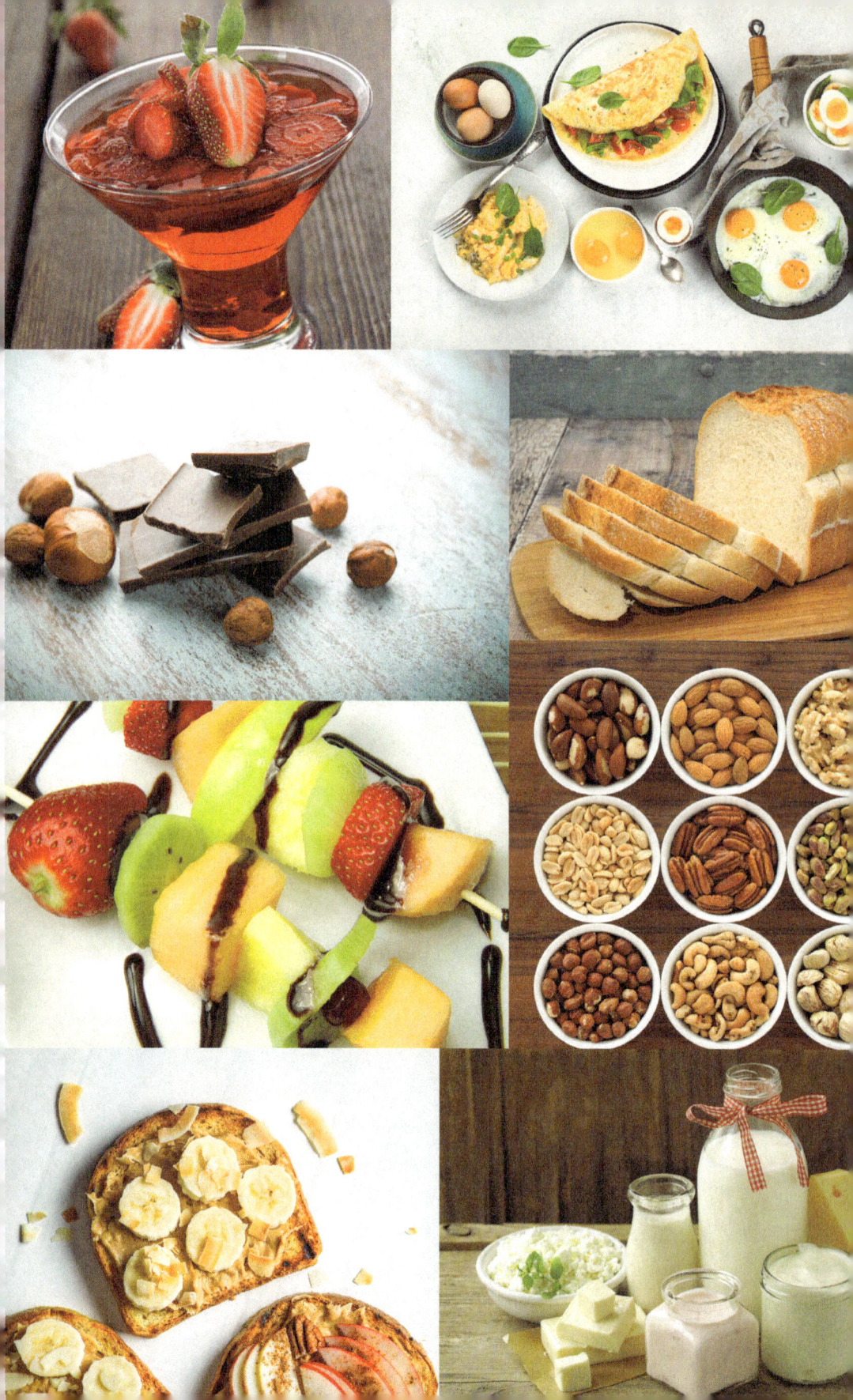

Simple 'Hacks' to Increase Good Nutrition

Myth: Starting a healthy diet as a senior citizen is too late.

It's never too late. Making an effort to change, decrease or delay the effects of poor nutrition can make a difference at any age.

1. Increase eating frequency.

In later years, we tend to feel less hungry, snack less often between the main meals, and have less cravings for food, in comparison to when we were younger. This is mostly due to changes in hormones to do with hunger. However, the less we eat, the less we get used to eating.

Encourage older people to eat three meals a day, plus snack regularly. Large plates of food can be intimidating and off putting. By making the portion size at meal time smaller and attractively presented, it will appear as less of a 'mountain to climb' and be more inviting.

Snacks can be healthy and attractive too. Making them as finger food means they are easy to eat and will be consumed less consciously.

a. Instead of sandwiches (where the majority of the portion is carbohydrate), put some delicious toppings on toast cut into really small, mouth sized, squares:

- Smashed avocado with a little smoked salmon
- Pate and a slice of olive
- Mashed / sliced banana with a drizzle of honey

- Nut butter with a slice of strawberry / banana
- Hummus
- Sliced egg
- Cream cheese and prawn
- Potted shrimps
- Mashed sardines with cream cheese

b. Portions of fruit with a twist (some might need a fork or cocktail stick):

- Apple slices and little squares of cheddar
- Apple slices sprinkled with honey or brown sugar
- Slice strawberries, grapes, kiwi, melon, banana, peaches, pears… with or without cocktail sticks… maybe with a tempting dip of melted dark chocolate or sweetened yoghurt
- Dried fruit with nuts and dark chocolate

c. Little pots of joy, eaten with a teaspoon:

- Prawn cocktail
- Apple puree with a dollop of cream
- Chocolate and avocado mousse *
- Full fat yoghurt
- Jelly with / without fruit
- Rice pudding with honey
- Ice cream with a granola / fruit topping
- Overnight oats *

2. Increase nutrient density.

To increase healthy calories, calcium, vitamins, and other minerals, it is very easy to upgrade staple food items, rather than increasing food intake.

a. Full fat milk, cream and cheese.

Not only are these delicious to most older people but they can add so much. All generations are now discovering that 'full fat'/'whole' milk is better than we have been led to believe. Full fat milk is far from full of fat:

   i. Regular/whole/full fat milk = 3.5% fat
   ii. Semi skimmed/low fat milk = 1.5% fat
   iii. Skimmed/fat free milk = 0.15% fat

Recent research has shown that there is little or no association between dairy fat and increased body fat [15].

Findings also indicated high-fat dairy consumption in a healthy diet doesn't contribute to heart disease or diabetes [16]. In fact, the findings of another study suggest greater dairy intake, especially full-fat dairy products, may actually decrease the risk of diabetes in middle-aged and older adults. Research also suggests that the combination of dairy amino acids, minerals, and fat is found to limit the effects of saturated fatty acids on blood cholesterol [17].

b. Eggs.

Not only is the tide turning on milk, but also on eggs. The British Heart Foundation and The Food Standards Agency have both scrapped their advice on limiting weekly egg consumption. Eggs are an incredible source of protein and Omega oil, and, just as importantly for the older generation, quick and easy to prepare.

The advice is to be careful about how it is cooked and what you eat it with. Fried eggs with bacon, sausage and white bread is obviously not a healthy meal. Soft boiled eggs are also not recommended if you have a weakened immune system.

- Scrambled eggs are the easiest, safest and quickest way to get good protein into an older person's diet. Mix it with full fat milk
- Sliced hard boiled egg on toast
- Baked eggs with mackerel and spinach *
- Spanish omelette
- Quiche *

c. Milk Powder.

Adding milk powder is the number 1 piece of advice I give to people. You can buy it in supermarkets under the trade name Marvel, or as own brand dried milk powder. It is usually skimmed (sadly) but you can buy full fat milk powder on the internet. (If you can only get skimmed, it will still add lots of protein and nutrients.)

My advice is to ignore the ratios on the packet when making it up. Take a few spoonfuls and mix it slowly with cold water or, better still, milk until it becomes a creamy texture. Then you can add it to anything 'creamy' to increase the protein level of things you normally eat.

Amount	Calories (kcals)	Protein (g)
1 pint semi skimmed milk	300	19.4
1 pint whole milk	396	19.2
1 pint whole milk with 4 tbsp dried whole milk powder	570	37.2

According to the West Suffolk NHS website [18]

You can add it to:

- Yoghurt
- Coffee and other milky drinks
- Custard
- Most puddings
- Curry
- Creamy sauces on chicken / fish etc
- Porridge

d. Nuts.

Nuts are an incredible source of protein, good fats and fibre. Almonds, walnuts, cashews, macadamia nuts and pistachios are all particularly good for people over 60. Other tree nuts are also nutritious… Brazil nuts, hazelnuts, pecans and pine nuts. Even peanuts (technically legumes) are full of protein, Omega-9 and carbohydrates.

A handful of any nuts (or a mixture) as a snack will really boost good nutrition.

Obviously, if chewing is an issue, you can buy them chopped, ground or even as 'butters'. Peanut, almond and cashew nut butters are all mainstream and readily available these days.

- Add a handful of mixed nuts to cereal
- Make your own granola
- Add ground nuts to savoury/sweet dishes
- Mix in with yoghurt, ice cream and fruit
- Add nut butter to soup or stir fries

- Put nuts or nut butter in crumble topping (apple and walnut etc.)
- Make nut butter ice cream*

*Recipe in Recipe Suggestions chapter

e. Nutritional Cakes.
At this point I have to mention Grandbar Snacks. These were created to be a healthy and delicious snack to help fight against weight loss. They are unbaked mini cakes made of oats (great fibre), with other natural sources of protein (nuts), Omega 3, prebiotics and antioxidants. Everything is finely ground, for anyone with chewing issues, with a layer of chocolate on the top.

f. Ready-Fortified Food.
Fortification is the deliberate addition of one or more macronutrient (ie: vitamins and minerals) with the aim of improving the health of the consumer.

I am not one, usually, to promote artificially added nutrients… but I concede that there might be a place for them.

i. Breakfast cereals

- *Kelloggs Cornflakes and Branflakes claim a 30g serving provides the average person with 25% of the Recommended Daily Allowance (RDA) of B Vitamins and 50% of the RDA of Vitamin D.*

- *Kelloggs Special K says a 30g serving provides between 30% to 50% of all B Vitamins, Vitamin D and Iron.*

- ***Weetabix says a 30g serving provides about 30% of some B Vitamins and Iron.***

- ***Nestle says that all its fortified cereals provide 15% or more of its listed vitamins and minerals in a 30g serving.***

ii. Bread

The Bread and Flour Regulations (1998) who control labelling and compositional standards for bread and flour specify that four vitamins and minerals must be added to all white and brown flour. These are calcium, iron, thiamine (Vitamin B1) and niacin (Vitamin B3).

In 2021, it became British law that Folic Acid had to be added to all white bread.

iii. Milk and Dairy Products

Milk is fortified with Vitamins A and D as standard in the USA. This is not the case in the UK. However, some producers have introduced fortified milk recently.

- Arla Big Milk has added Iron, Vitamin A and Vitamin D
- ASDA has a Vitamin D milk range

Yoghurts are more commonly fortified with pro and pre biotics, as well as protein.

Probiotics are live bacteria and yeast that are thought, by some, to replace those lost with poor diets and antibiotics.

- ***Actimel, Yakult and Activia are the most common yoghurts with probiotics***

Prebiotics are slightly better, in that they feed the microbiomes in your gut, so they are stronger and reproduce. Most prebiotics are found in very fibrous food… which is not great in old age. However, they are often added to yoghurts and other snacks.

- ***Look for yoghurts with ingredients such as inulin, lactulose and chicory root, as well as honey.***

g. Oral Nutritional Supplements

When someone is really weak from illness or frailty, and eating solid food is really not an option, there are products designed just for this problem. The Community Nurse or GP might recommend they have a nutrition drink. These are mostly made of water and milk protein, and fortified with minerals and vitamins, high in calories and fibre.

- ***Ensure, Fortisip and Huel are the main makes.***
- ***Complan is a more traditional brand that you can buy in powder form and make up yourself.***

Recipe Suggestions

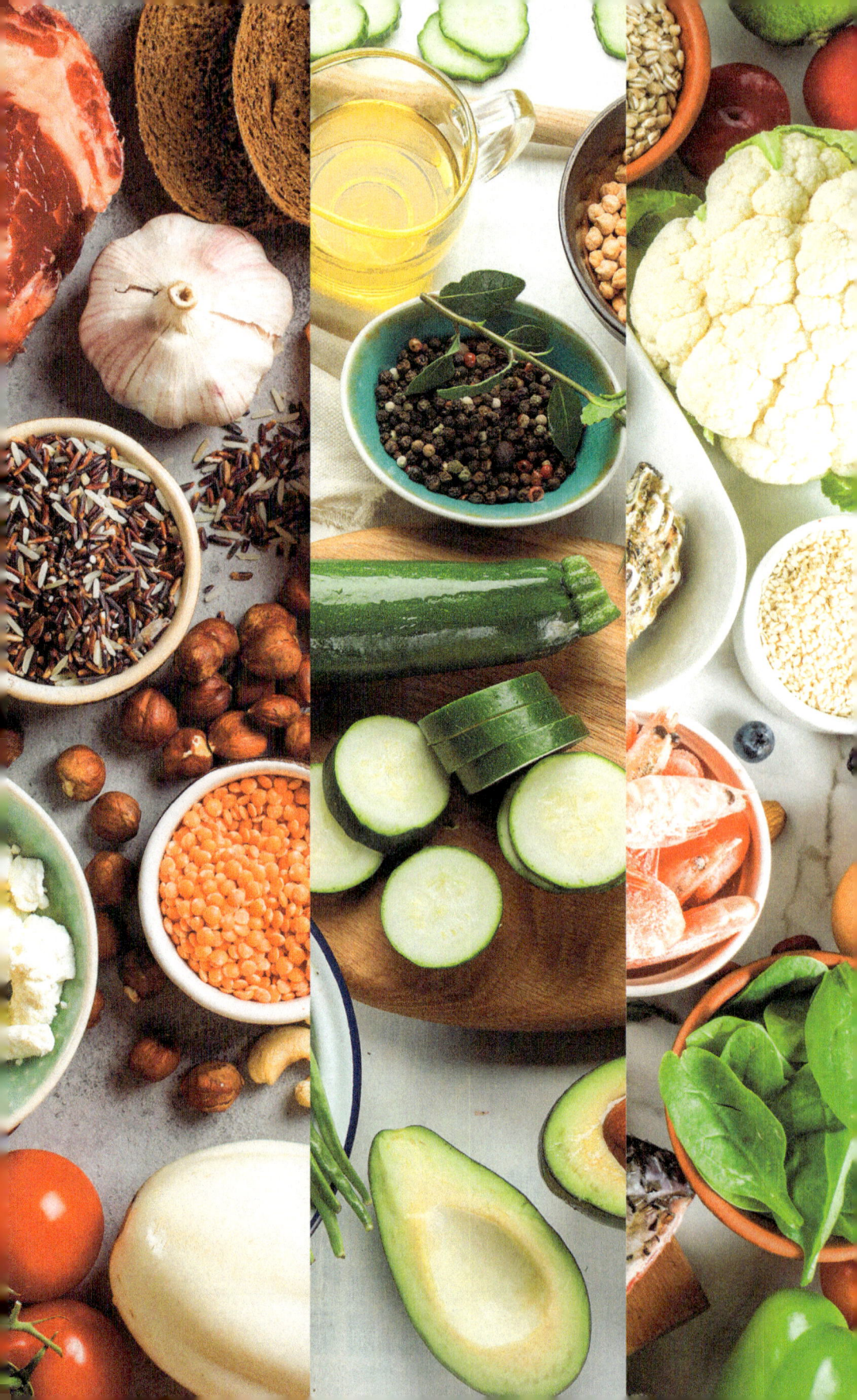

Recipe Suggestions

Myth: Easy to eat soft food loses its nutrients, tastes bland and is boring to eat.

Absolutely not. There is no need to overcook or boil healthy food in order for it to be easy to eat.

Breakfast

1. Overnight Oats.

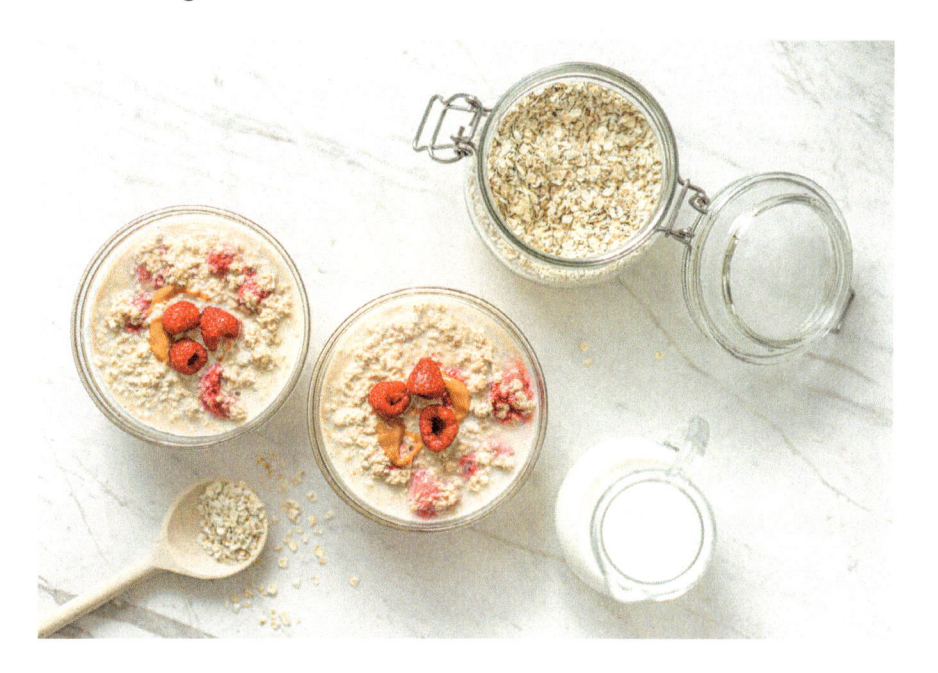

These are the loveliest and easiest thing to make:

> 30g of any oats. If you need something smooth then Readybrek is probably your best bet.
> 1 tub of yoghurt. Any flavour you like but FULL FAT and preferably with prebiotics.

Couple of spoonfuls of dried milk powder.
Any fruit you want to add (I love adding a banana and about 4 frozen strawberries).
Teaspoonful of nut butter.

Mix it all together in a bowl or plastic tub. Put the lid on and leave overnight in the fridge. By morning you'll have a delicious breakfast (I make 2 or 3 at once so I have a few days' worth).

2. Scrambled eggs / omelette.

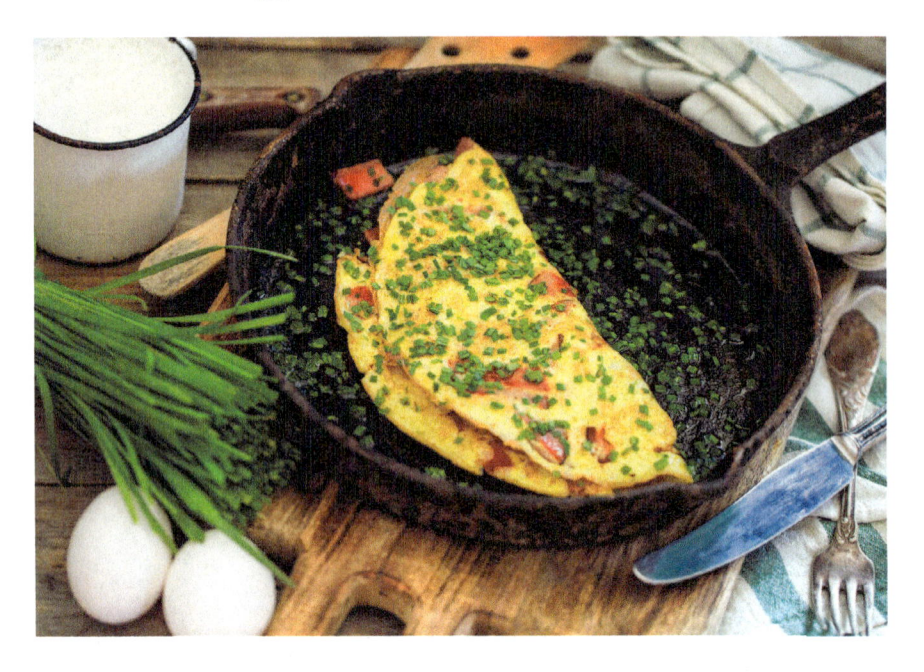

The great things about eggs are that they are easy to get hold of, not too expensive and really easy to cook! There's no weekly minimum advised any more – its what you eat with them that can be the unhealthy bit.

- Make your scrambled eggs with full fat milk (mixed with some dried milk powder).

Serve with avocado, wilted spinach and / or smoked salmon to add extra nutrition.

- Omelettes can have almost anything added... chopped onions, peppers, tomatoes, mushrooms, spinach, ham, mackerel, avocado – you name it! Add lots of cheese to pack in the calories and calcium.

3. Banana pancakes.

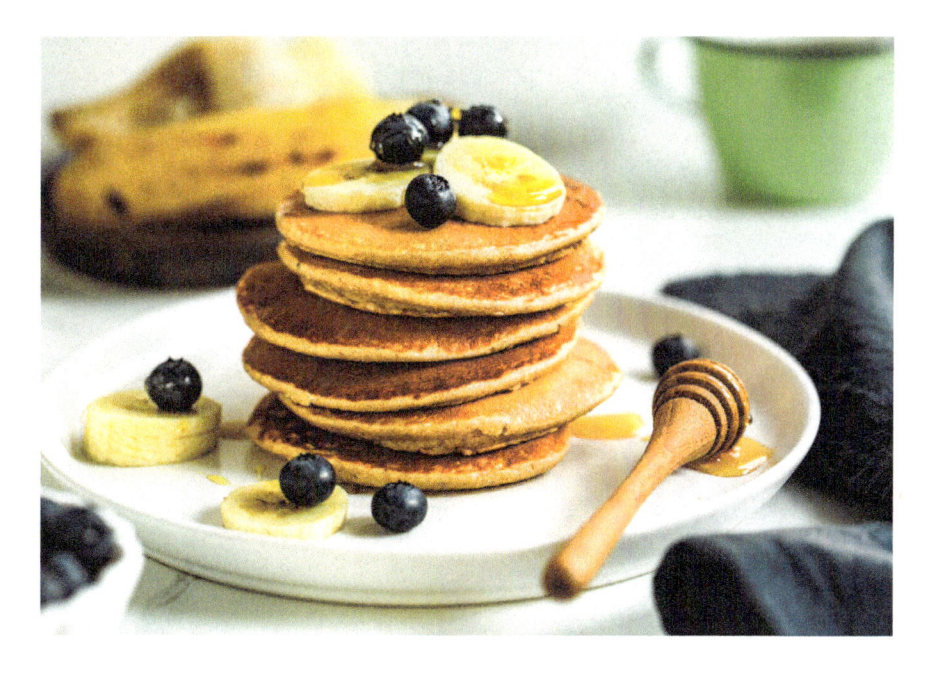

Really easy and much more nutritious than traditional English or American pancakes.

The SIMPLEST recipe is as follows:

    1 banana (ripe)
    1 heaped tablespoon self raising flour
    ½ teaspoon baking powder

1 egg
Pinch of salt
Splash of vanilla extract
(you could add spinach or oats too)

Mix all the ingredients in a blender for 20 seconds. Pour 3 to 4 little pools of mixture into an oiled and heated frying pan. Turn them over after a minute, or when they are starting to bubble. Fry on the other side for about 30 seconds.

Serve with fruit, yoghurt, thick cream or maple syrup.

There are plenty of fancier recipes on the internet if you want to upgrade your breakfast experience!

Lightish Lunch

1. Crustless Quiche.

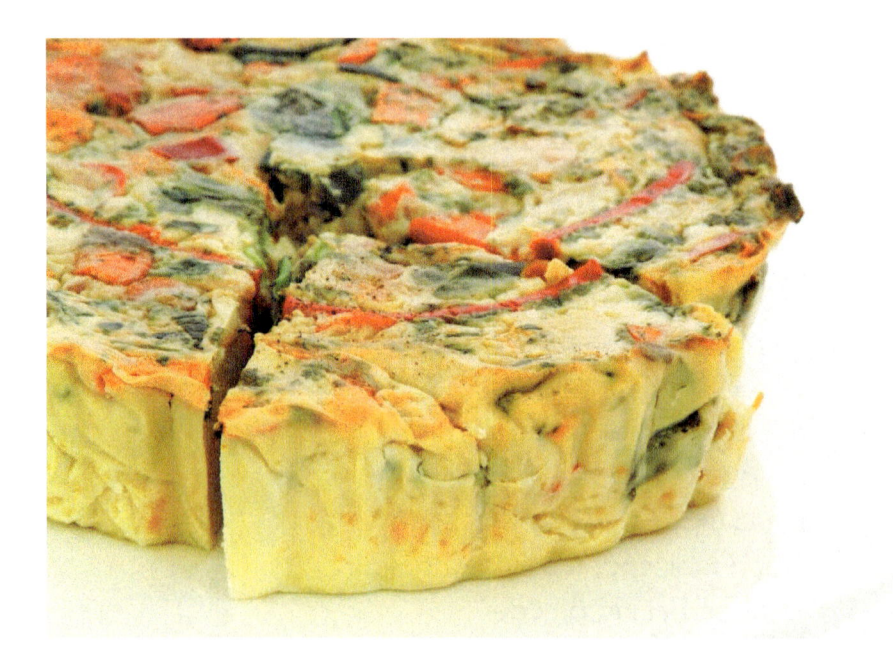

I tend to make pastry-free quiche. As with everything I suggest, when appetite is low try not to fill up on 'empty calories'. Hence the lack of pastry.

Preheat oven to 180'C, Fan 160'C, Gas mark 4

300ml pot double cream
100ml full fat milk
3 eggs
140g grated cheddar cheese

Suggestions for filling:
- Goats cheese
- Cubed ham
- Onions
- Mushrooms
- Asparagus
- Herbs
- Salmon
- Feta
- Spinach
- Tomatoes
- Butternut squash
- Courgettes
- Leeks
- Artichokes
- Broad beans
- Peas
- Peppers
- Prawns

Precook any of the fillings that might need frying / boiling first.

Line a flan dish / baking tray with parchment or a baking sheet and grease with butter or spray with oil.

Whisk the cream, milk, eggs and cheese together, add the filling to the mix, then turn into the lined, greased dish.

Bake in the oven for 20 – 30 minutes until golden brown.

2. Fish cakes.

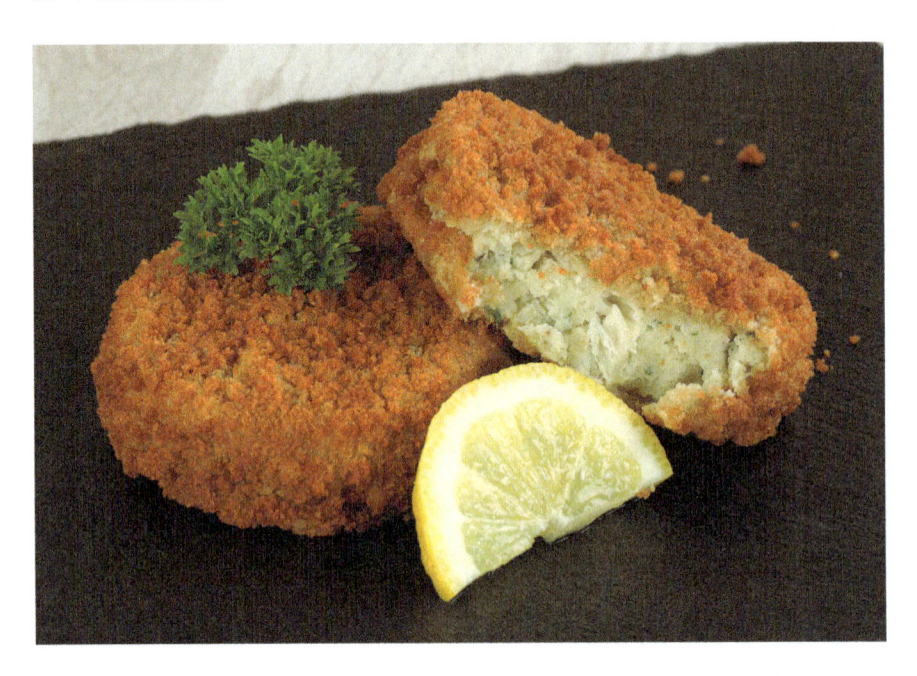

Another great recipe that can be as simple or fancy as you wish. I will give you the very easiest version I can come up with!

    1 (300 – 400g) pack fish pie mix, or any fish
    400g supermarket chilled mashed potato / frozen mash / packet of instant mash (made up with milk or water)
    Couple of spoons of milk powder
    1 tablespoon of cream cheese, double cream or crème

fraiche (or an egg)
Salt and pepper
Flour

If you like, add:
- Spring onions
- Parsley
- Garlic
- Egg and breadcrumbs

Steam or poach the fish. Mix the fish, mash, cream cheese (or alternative), milk powder, salt and pepper with a fork. Mix well as the more you work it the less likely the fish cake will collapse when cooking.

Either just dip in flour and fry, or, if you prefer, dip in flour, egg and breadcrumbs and then fry.

3. Hearty Soup.

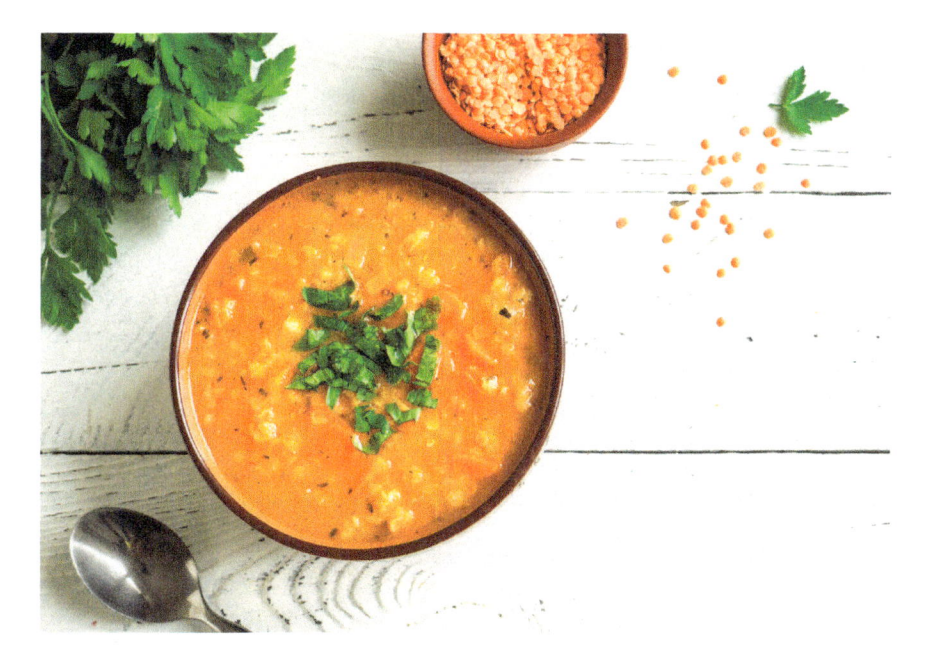

Soup can be as thick or thin as prefered. A whole meal in a bowl!

This recipe makes 6-8 portions, so ideal to make and freeze.

900g chicken or Quorn pieces

And roughly:
1 onion
4 celery sticks
3 carrots
1 large potato
½ butternut squash

Plus if you like:
- Mushrooms
- Tinned chickpeas, lentils, mixed beans
- Cabbage
- Courgette
- Pasta
- Pearl barley (a favourite of mine)
- Garlic

1.4 litre hot chicken or vegetable stock
3 tablespoons normal strength tomato puree
1 teaspoon Italian seasoning
1 teaspoon garlic powder
Salt and pepper
1 tablespoon olive oil

Brown chicken and then the chopped vegetables in the olive oil. Put ALL ingredients in a saucepan, crockpot or slow cooker.

Cook well. 30-40+ minutes on the hob, or (preferably) a few hours / overnight in the slow cooker.

Either shred the chicken before serving, or let it cool slightly, and blitz it in a blender or with a hand blender.

4. Baked eggs with mackerel and spinach.

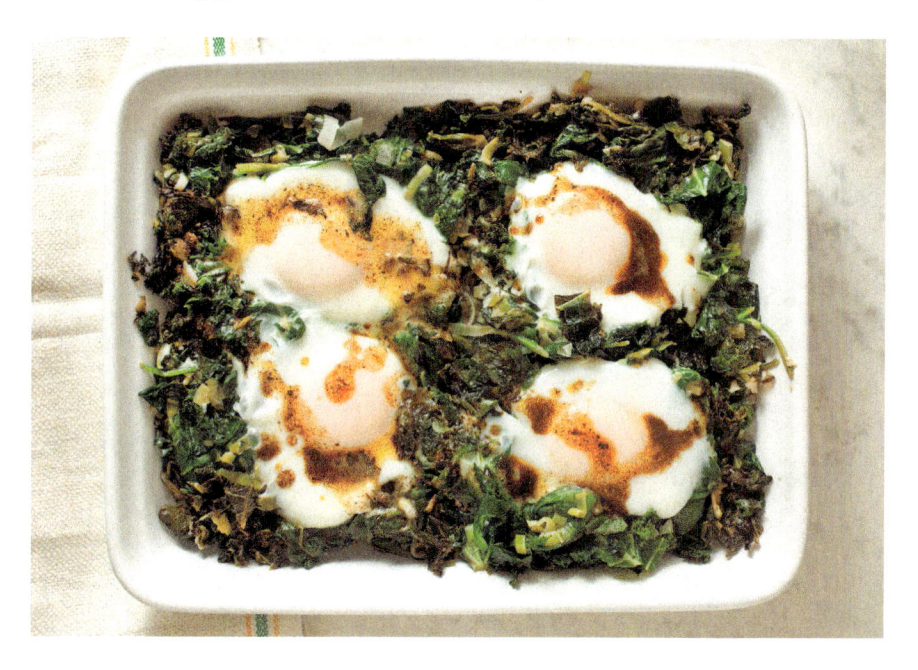

This recipe serves 4, so adjust if necessary.

Preheat oven to 200'C, Fan 180'C or Gas Mark 6

    8 eggs
    200mg mackerel with skin removed
    1 teaspoon horseradish sauce
    200g spinach
    3 tablespoons crème fraiche
    Herbs such as chives, parsley or coriander

Wilt spinach by putting it in a colander and pouring boiling water over. When cooled, squeeze out all excess water and divide into 4 dishes, or just the one.

Separately mix the crème fraiche with the herbs and horseradish. Flake the mackerel and add, then place mixture on top of the spinach.

Crack 2 eggs in each small dish, or all 8 into the larger one. Cover each dish with foil. Bake for 15 minutes.

Remove and leave to stand for 2 minutes before serving.

Snacks

There's a list of simple snacks in the previous chapter, but here's a few more:

1. Cheesy Courgette Muffins.

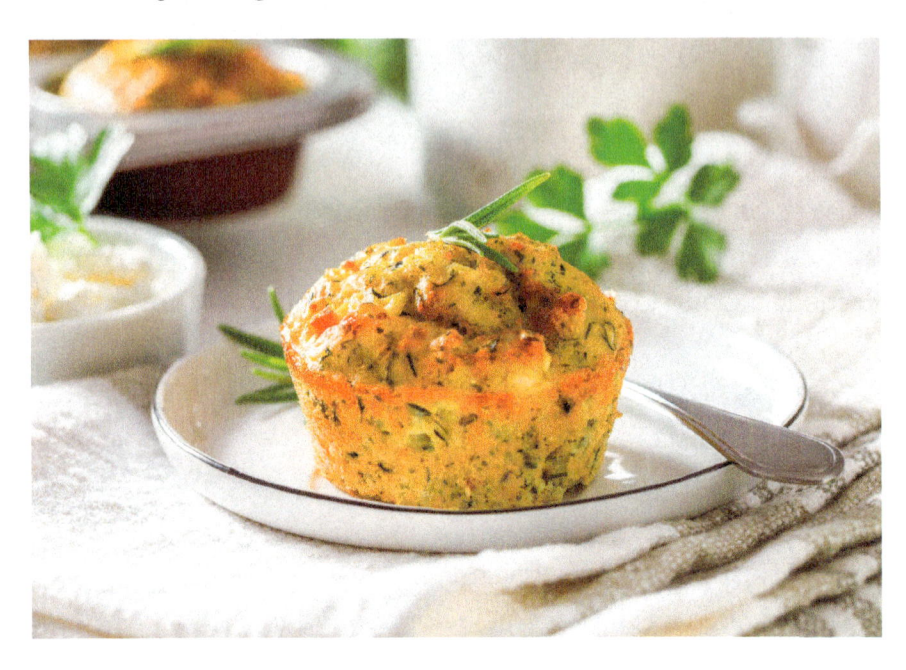

This recipe makes 12 small muffins which can be frozen.

Preheat oven to 200'C, Fan 180'C or Gas Mark 6

> 1 courgette or 80g peas
> 100g cheddar cheese
> 225g self raising flour
> 50ml olive oil
> 175ml full fat milk
> 1 egg
> Black pepper

Grate the courgette and the cheese. Mix all the ingredients together gently in a bowl.

Cook in the oven for about 20 minutes until golden brown.

2. Nut Butter Brownies.

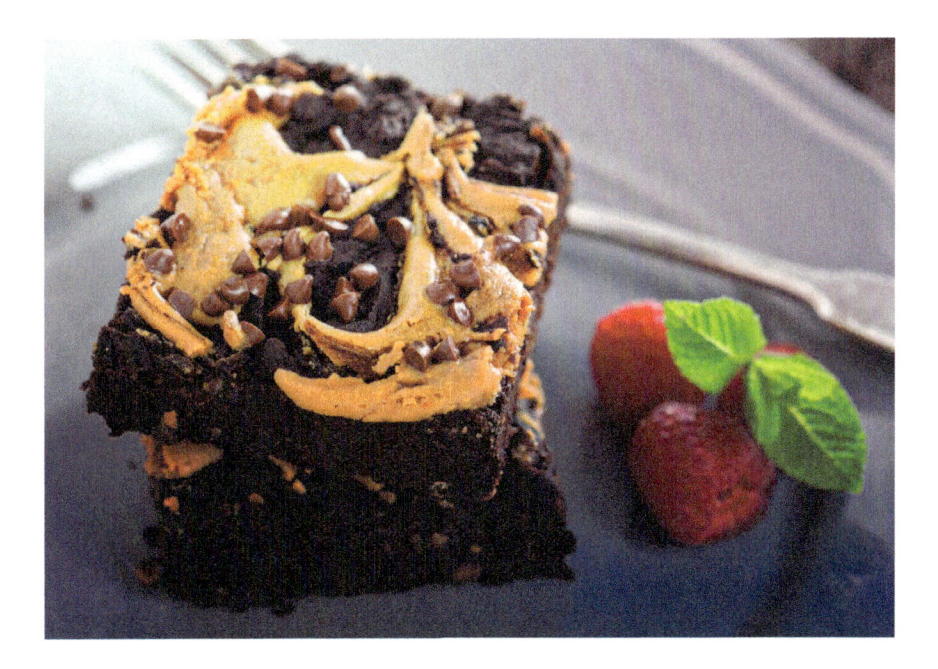

For the chocoholics! Makes 16 squares.

Preheat oven to 180'C, Fan 160'C Gas Mark 4

    175g nut butter (almond, hazlenut, cashew etc.)
    150g dark chocolate
    280g soft light brown sugar
    3 eggs
    100g self raising flour

Gently melt the nut butter, chocolate and sugar in a pan, stirring occasionally. When done, put into a bowl to cool slightly.

Beat in the eggs one at a time with a wooden spoon, then fold in the flour.

Turn into a 20cm square baking tray that you've lined with baking parchment.

Cook in the oven for 20 – 25 minutes (until the top is crusty but the inside is still a bit sticky).

If you fancy, you could drizzle an extra 50g of melted chocolate on the top and then cool in the tin before cutting up.

3. Apple Crumble Bites.

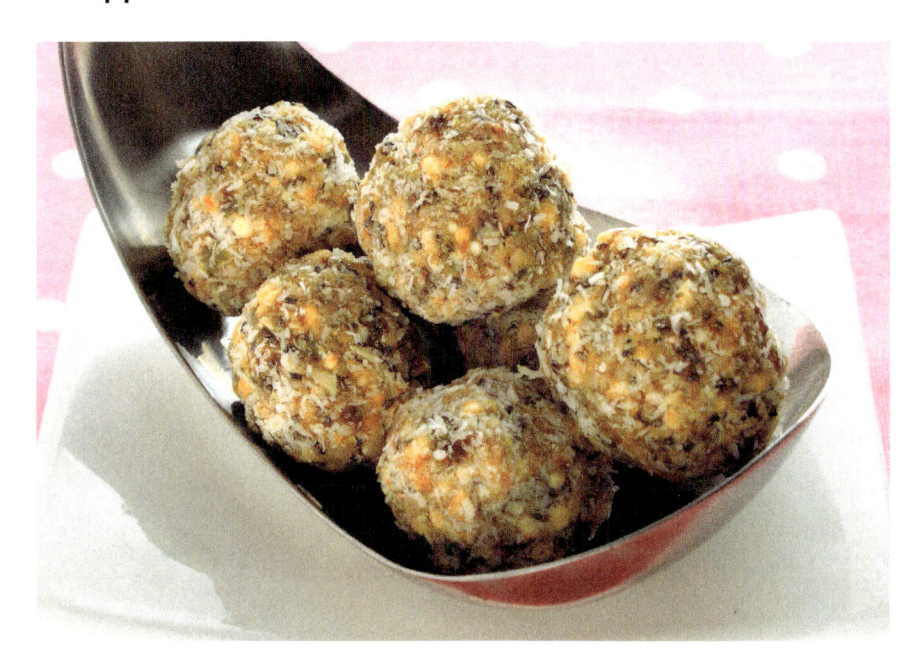

Full of great nutrition and really delicious. Eat with chunks of cheese perhaps?

    50g oats
    50g pitted dates
    2 tablespoons of almond (or any nut) butter
    50g ground, chopped or whole almonds
    ¼ teaspoon cinnamon
    30g dried apple slices (from most supermarkets or health food stores)
    ½ apple
    Pinch of salt
    White chocolate

Mix 30g of oats and the dates, almond butter, almonds, cinnamon, salt and apple slices in a blender until smooth. Grate up the apple (including the skin if you wish), then add that and the rest of the oats to the mixture and blitz again.

Form into about 10 balls… or any shape that's easy to eat. Put on parchment and cool in the fridge. Then melt the white chocolate and dip each piece in before returning to the fridge to harden. They should last about a week.

Main Meals

If you ensure that the meals are made up of foods that provide multiple nutrient sources, then you will know that every mouthful is beneficial. For example:

1. Salmon with sweet potato mash and broccoli.

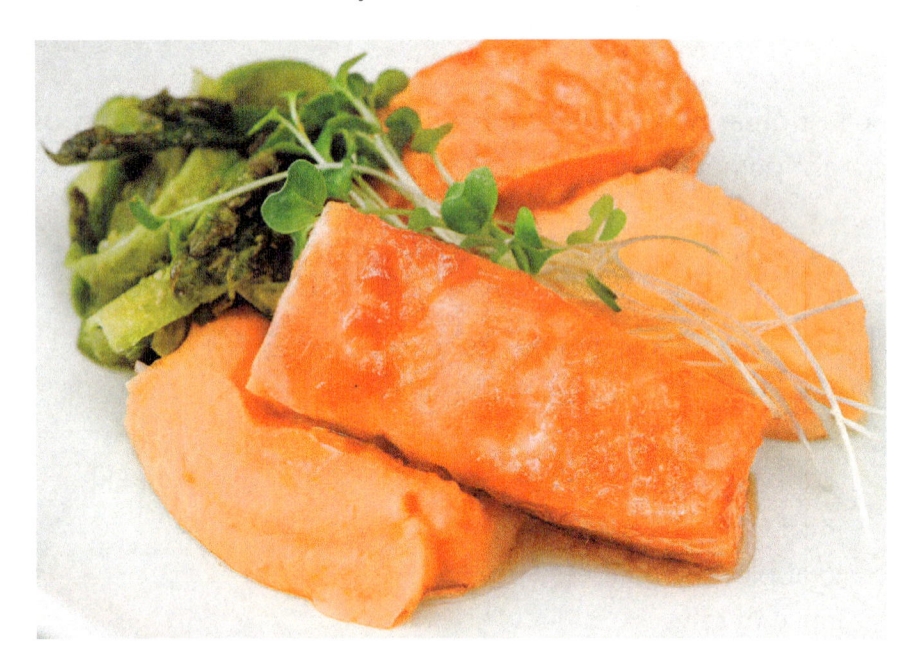

A quick trick… chop the sweet potato into wedges (skins still on), put in a bowl with a desert spoon of water, cover and microwave on full power for about 15 minutes. Meanwhile poach / steam the salmon and broccoli for the same amount of time. You can now easily remove the skin and mash the sweet potato with butter, milk and cheese.

2. Chilli with lots of vegetables.

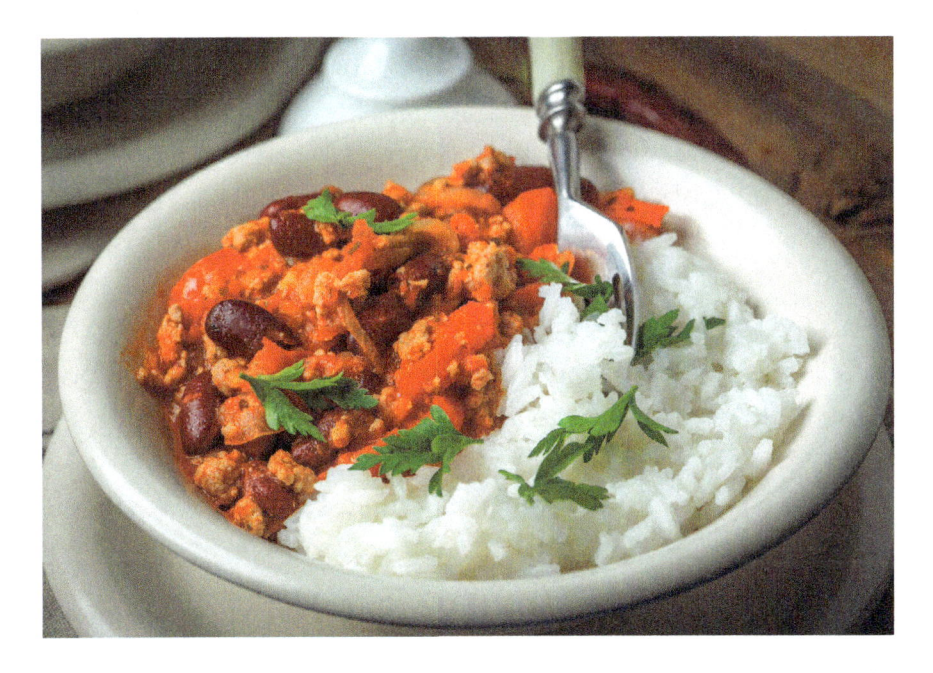

Chilli doesn't have to be spicy and I've discovered a fabulous recipe which means you just chuck everything in the slow cooker, with no need to brown first.

500g lean beef mince (As all the fat will stay in the dish, it's best to use the 5% type. If you prefer to use higher fat mince, it is best to brown it first and drain it.) or 500g Quorn mince

    1 onion or 200g ready chopped / frozen onion
    Tin chopped tomatoes
    Tin red kidney beans
    3 tablespoons normal strength tomato puree

300g mushrooms
1 red pepper
1 large carrot
4 celery sticks
1 or 2 beef (or vegetable) stock cubes
1 teaspoon cumin (or to taste)
1 teaspoon cayenne / mild / strong chilli powder (whichever you prefer)
1 teaspoon garlic powder or granules
20g Dark Chocolate (70%)
200g full fat crème fraiche or plain yoghurt

Chop the vegetables (or use ready chopped / frozen veg) and put all the ingredients into the slow cooker. Cook on high for 6 hours, or low for 8. Stir occasionally to break up the mince.

Serve on a jacket potato or rice with the crème fraiche / yoghurt

3. Lentil cottage pie (with cheese topping).

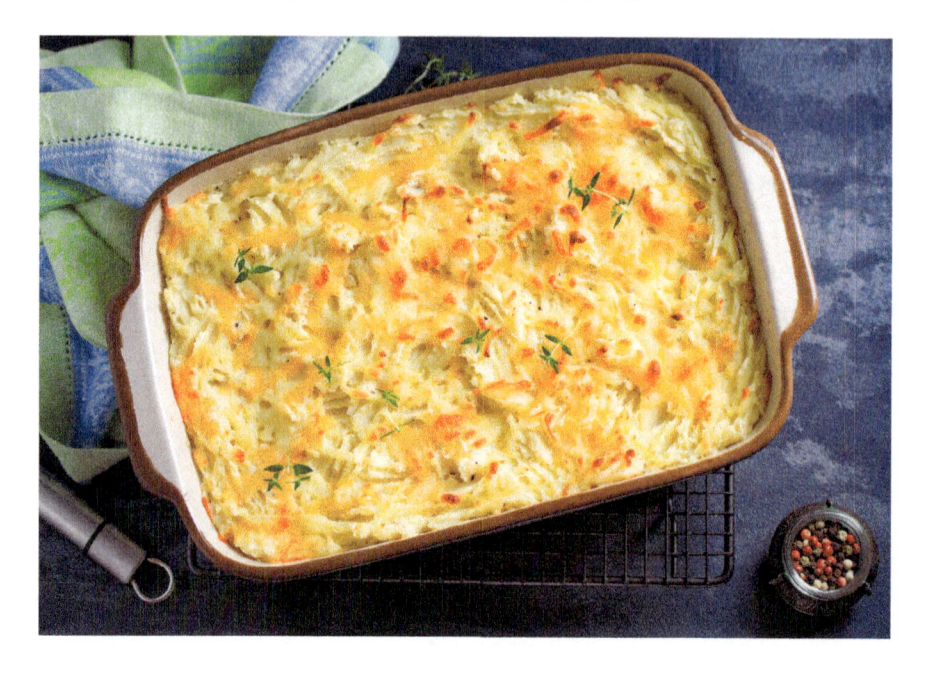

Delicious, healthy and another simple recipe.

Preheat oven to 220'C, Fan 200'C or Gas Mark 7.
- 200g dried green lentils
- 25g butter
- 1 leek
- 150g mushrooms
- 2 carrots
- 2 cloves of garlic (crushed or grated)
- 2 tins chopped tomatoes
- 200ml water
- 1 Vegetable stock cube
- Worcestershire Sauce or soy sauce to taste

For the topping:
- 400g supermarket chilled mashed potato
- Or frozen mash
- Or packet of instant mash (made up with milk or water)
- 50ml double cream
- 75g cheddar cheese

Fry leeks on low for a few minutes, then add the mushrooms and garlic until starting to brown.

Add all the other filling ingredients and simmer on the hob for 25 minutes.

Mix mashed potato with cream and 50g cheese.

Place filling in a large ovenproof dish and top with the mash mix. Sprinkle over the 25g of cheese and bake for 15 – 20 minutes.

Serve alone or with extra vegetables like peas or cabbage.

Of course, you can use tinned beans or lentils, but just use the water from the can instead of the 200ml.

Desserts

1. Chocolate and avocado mousse.

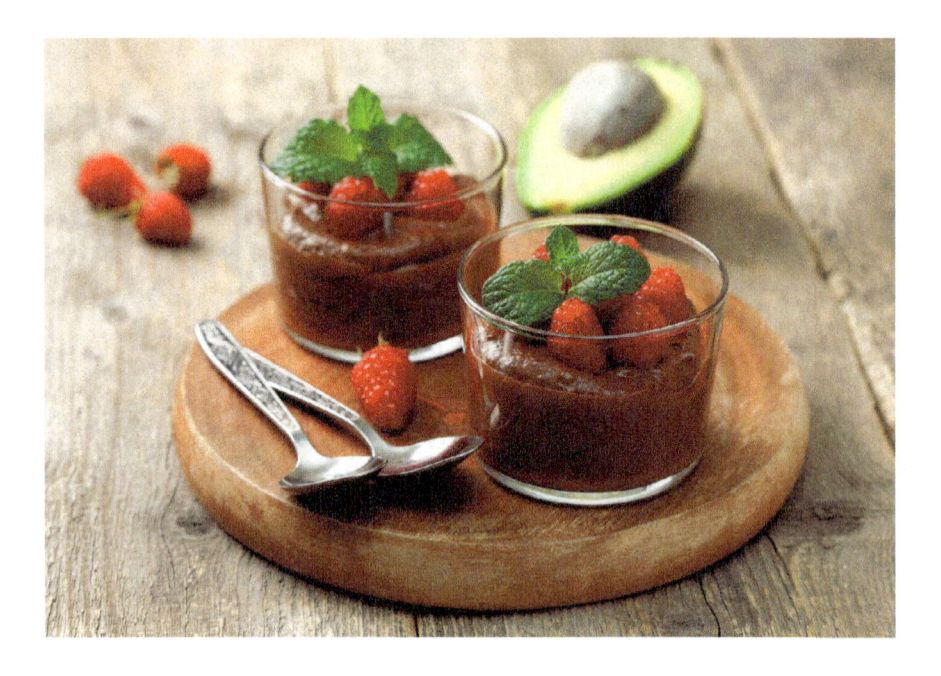

A strange sounding mix, but you can't taste the avocado….it's actually delicious and full of goodness!

> 2 ripe avocados
> 40g cocoa powder
> 40g melted dark chocolate (70%)
> 2 tablespoons full fat milk
> 2 tablespoons double cream (or 4 tablespoons of non dairy milk)

1 teaspoon vanilla essence
60ml honey / maple syrup or agave syrup
Pinch of salt

After melting the chocolate, mix all the ingredients in a blender until smooth.

Put into serving dishes and chill for 3 to 12 hours.

2. Nut butter icecream.

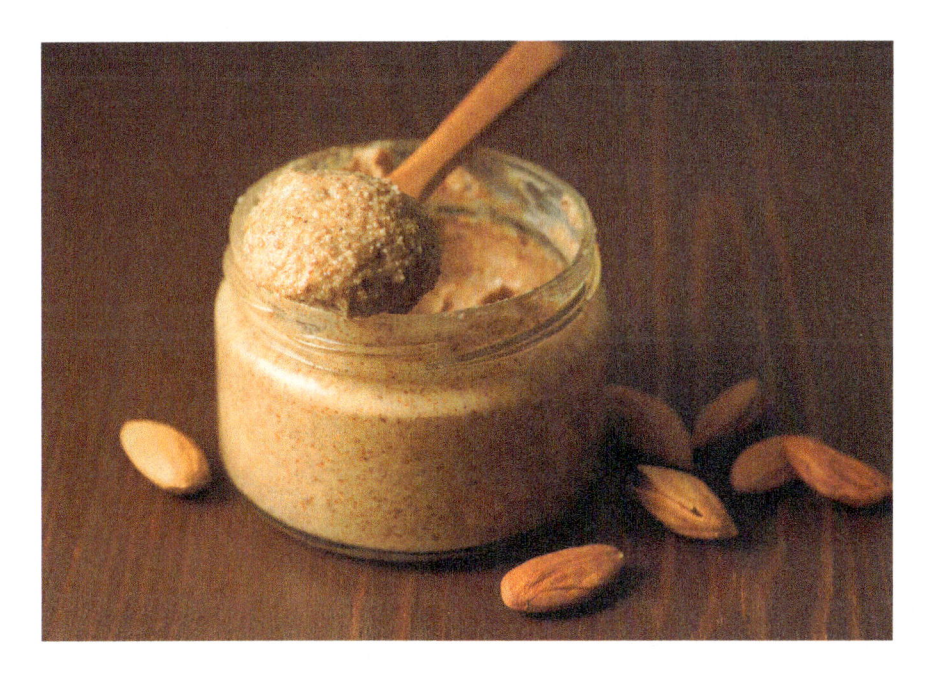

Full of really nutritious calories and so delicious!

1 can condensed milk
360g of nut butter… peanut or almond butter
500ml double cream (chilled)
1 teaspoon vanilla extract
180g dark chocolate (70%) broken into small pieces

Mix the condensed milk and 280g of nut butter in a large bowl.

Melt the rest of the nut butter in the microwave in 30 second 'bursts' until quite runny.

In an electric mixer whisk the cream and vanilla until stiff peaks form. Fold this, and the dark chocolate into the nut and condensed milk mixture.

Turn this into a container while drizzling in the runny nut butter. Cover tightly with clingfilm, put the container lid on and freeze for at least 6 hours.

3. Crumble.

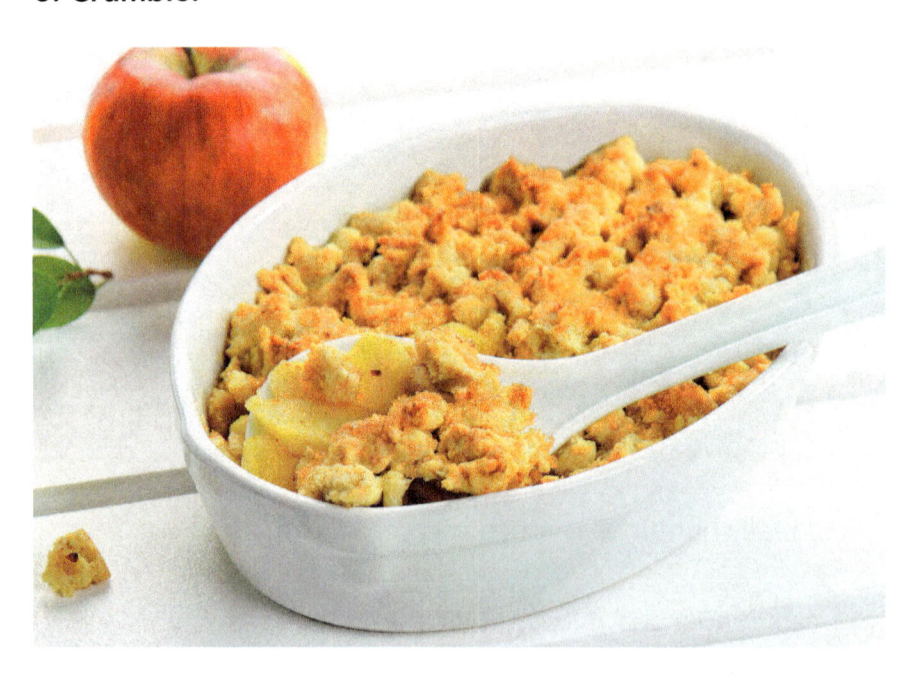

You can't beat a crumble for good old fashioned warming food, that can take a whole load of healthy 'beefing up'!

Preheat oven to 200'C, Fan 180'C or Gas Mark 6

> 1 or 2 eating apples
> 500g frozen fruit (mixed berries or anything that takes your fancy)
> 80g soft brown sugar
> 50g of nut butter or butter (or half and half)
> 20g oats
> 20g mixed chopped nuts
> 70g flour

Add cinnamon or ginger, if you fancy.

Put the frozen fruit into a large bowl, cover and put in the microwave on high for 10 minutes until defrosted (or overnight in the fridge). Drain the juice. Peel, core and thinly slice the apples.

Put the apples in with the berries and half the sugar. Mix well and then place it all in an oven dish.

In a mixing bowl, rub / stir the nut butter (and butter) together with the flour, then add the oats, nuts and the rest of the sugar.

Place the crumble topping on top of the fruit and bake for 25 minutes or until golden brown.

Serve with nut ice cream or custard (made with full fat milk and added dried milk!).

Hydration

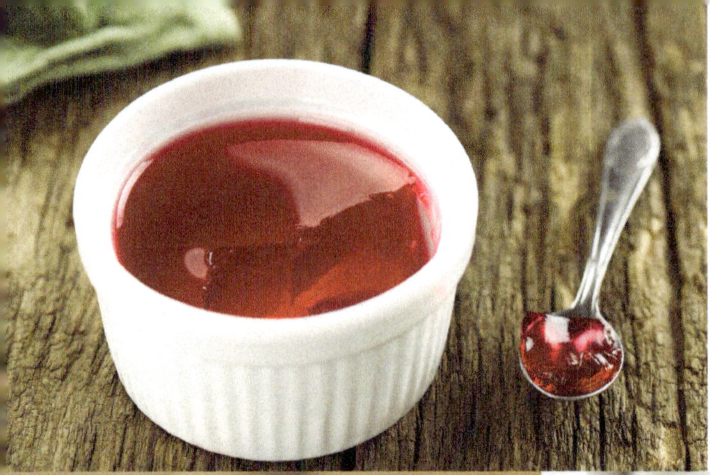
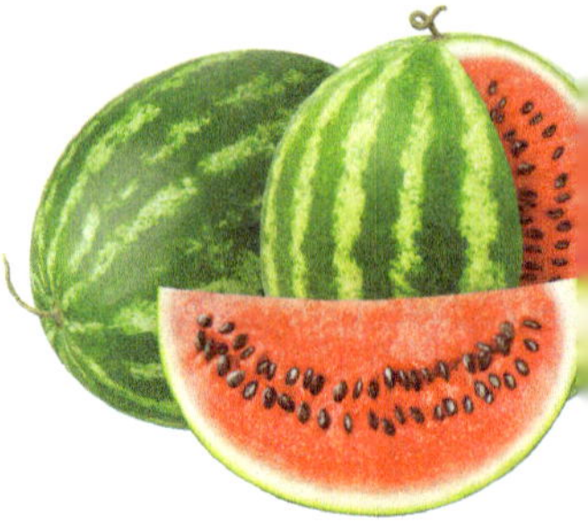
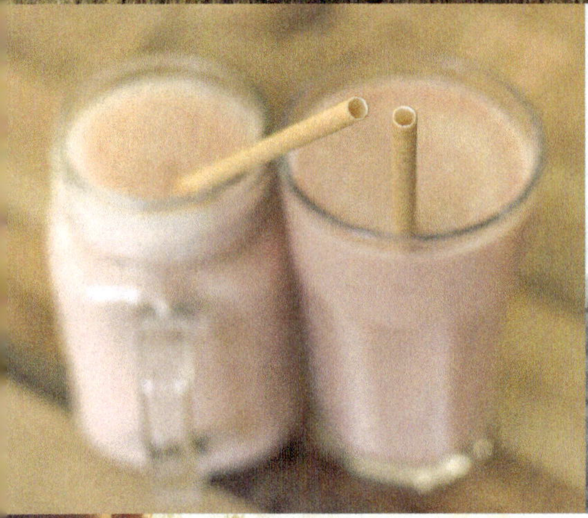
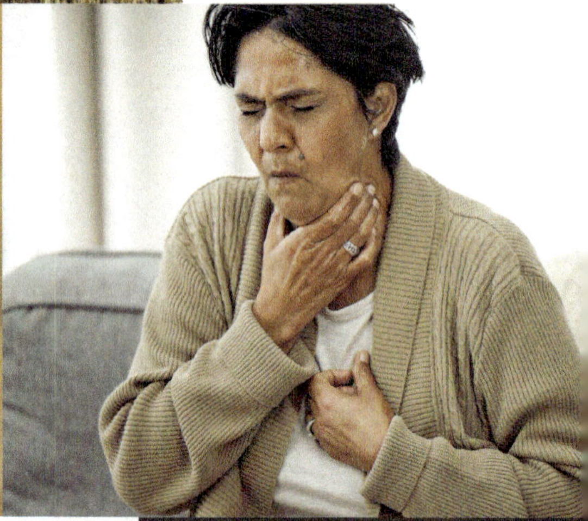
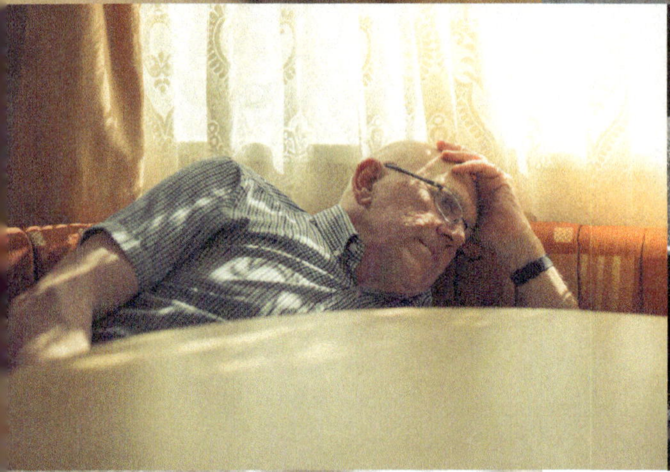
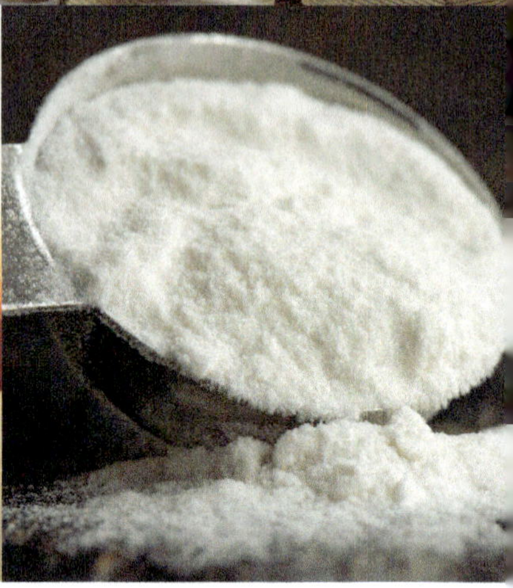
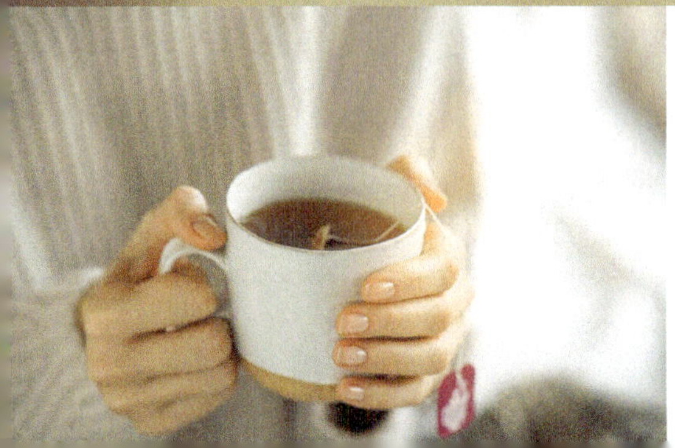
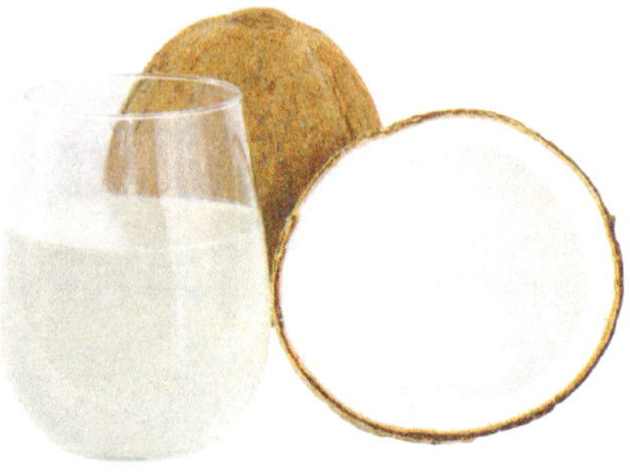

Hydration

Myth: Only water stops dehydration. You must have 6 – 8 drinks a day (1.2 litres). Caffeinated drinks don't count.

Not true. Liquid is found in all sorts of foods and drinks. Fruits and vegetables are excellent sources of water, and tea and coffee do count (the diuretic effect does not offset hydration) [19].

As well as struggling to eat enough, not drinking enough is also often a massive issue. In fact, we need to drink MORE as we get older to help our weaker kidneys.

The problems/reasons:

- Lack of desire to get out of your chair to go to the kitchen to make a drink / depression
- Reduced sensation of thirst
- Worrying about incontinence or 'accidents'
- Carrying, holding or drinking from a mug or cup can be tricky
- Fear of 'it going down the wrong way' because of decreased strength in swallowing
- Being in a care home or hospital with poor quality care
- Diuretics and laxatives
- And many more

The impacts:

- Urinary tract infections, acute kidney injury
- Constipation

- Low blood pressure, light headedness
- Tiredness, poor concentration
- Pressure sores and skin conditions
- Twice as likely to die if you have a stroke

Some Solutions:

- Pureed fruit, yoghurts, gravy, soup, ice cream and custard all are liquids
- Jelly is one of the best ways of getting liquid if drinking is an issue
- Coconut water is amazing as it also provides natural electrolytes, but it's important to sip it, not gulp it down as it can cause bloating
- Watermelon and all melons are extremely high in water
- Sugary drinks like cola or energy drinks (plus rehydration sachets) can help in acute situations as a short term solution to dehydration

For people with really weak swallowing, there are starch based thickeners you can buy and add to any drink. Even if someone can't hold the cup or drink safely, they can still enjoy 'a nice cuppa tea'!

Straws and sippy cups are quite useful, simple ideas too.

Helping someone to eat

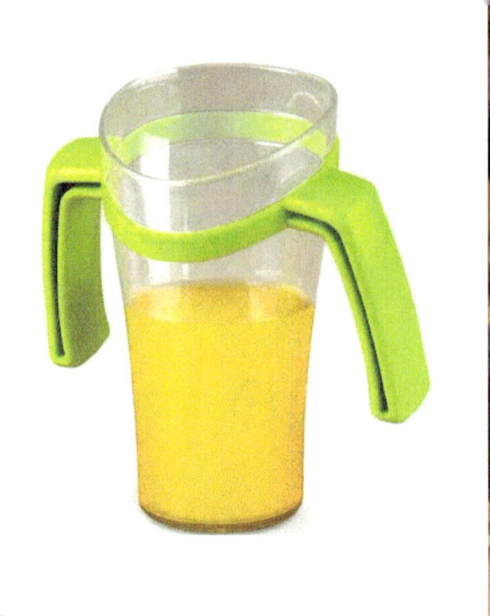
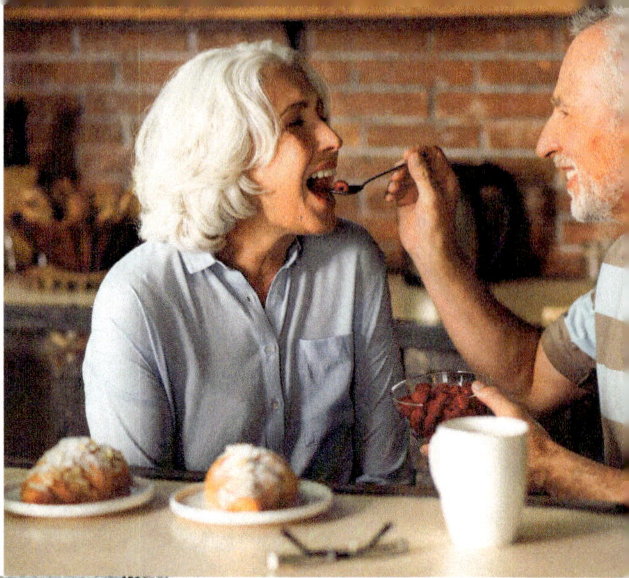
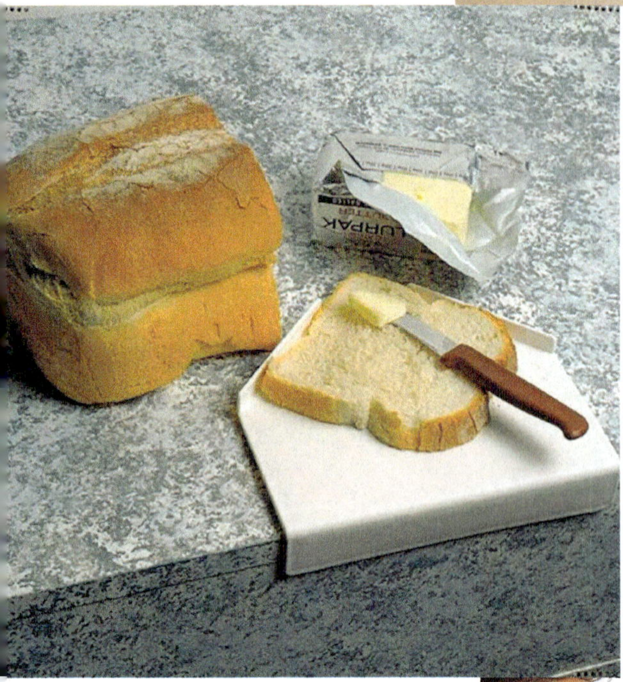
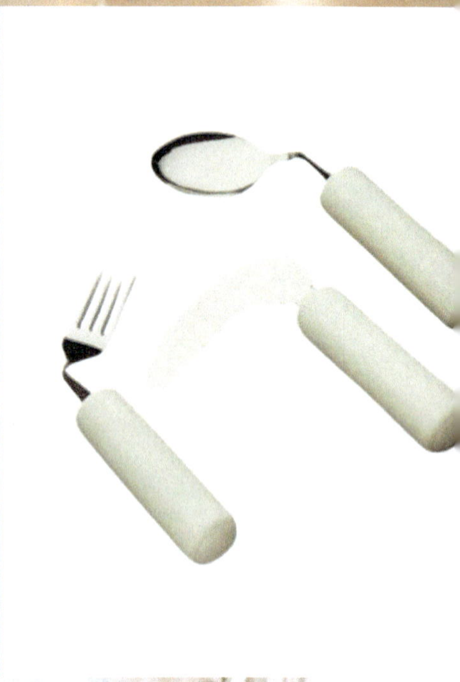
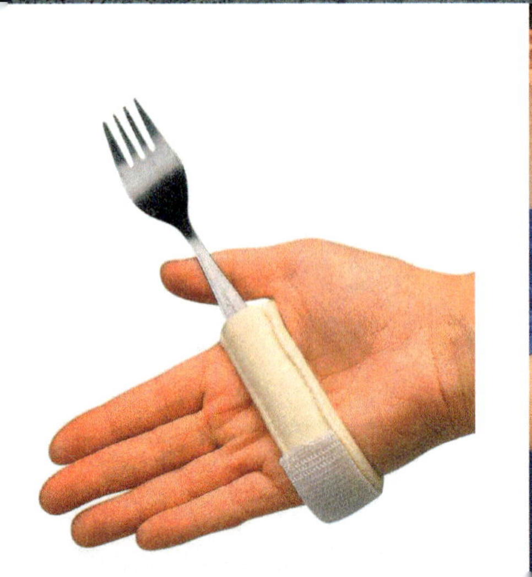
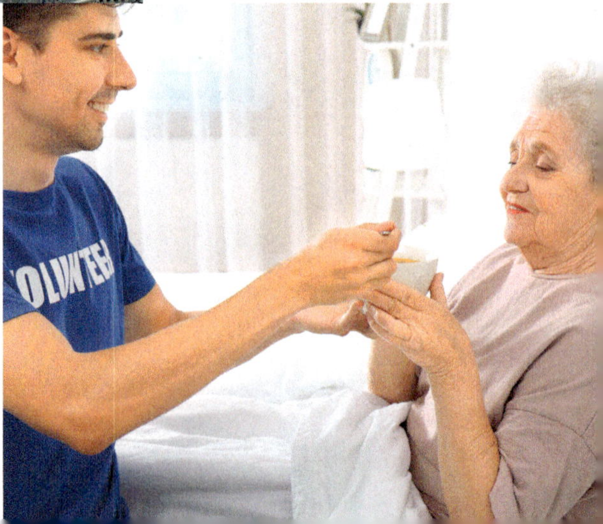

Helping someone to eat

There may come a time when you or someone may need help with eating. This may be due to muscle weakness, neurological disorder or dementia.

1. Equipment.
Thankfully there is plenty of adapted equipment to help you eat and drink more effectively and independently.

There are special cups that:

- Have two handles
- Are sloped already, so you don't have to twist your wrists so much
- Are weighted differently
- Have spouts
- Have lids
- Keep drinks warm for longer

There is cutlery with:

- Soft grip handles
- Angled handles
- Straps, so they don't drop out of your hand

There are angled plates and plate guards, as well as lots of kitchen aids, such as:

- Talking kitchen scales
- Chopping boards / work stations
- Keep warm plates / bowls

- Non slip mats
- Easy open containers
- Safe sharp knives

These can be found on many healthcare or shopping sites on the internet.

2. Prompting and assisting.

While it is best that everyone is encouraged to eat independently, if they can, some people may still need support. They may need you to hold a fork or spoon to the mouth.

- *Always think of it as helping someone to eat, rather than 'feeding' them. It's all about keeping their dignity and control.*

- *Make it a happy / social experience, rather than a chore. Engage with them fully.*

- *Give cues about meal time. Lay a setting in front of them and let them smell it first. Gently stroking someone's arm might give them a clue that it's meal time.*

- *Make sure you are both sitting comfortably:*
    - *Ensure their glasses, dentures and / or hearing aids are on and comfortable*
    - *The person should be sitting as upright as possible*
    - *You should sit facing the person you are assisting and at their level or slightly lower*

- *Communication.*
    - *Maintain comfortable eye contact.*
    - *Smile.*
    - *Talk about the food. Tell them what it is (if it's pureed its not always easy to tell!). Describe the food and give options using a gentle tone. Even if it's just 'would you like some potato next?'*
    - *Use phrases like "this looks tasty" to keep them focused and encouraged.*
    - *Don't ask questions or tell a joke... their reaction may cause choking!*
    - *Give verbal prompts like "open your mouth please" or "remember to chew".*

- *Eating*
    - *Touching their lips with the food might make them open their mouth.*
    - *Give small mouthfuls, but enough for them to feel the food in their mouth.*
    - *Give enough time to chew and swallow before offering more. Don't rush.*
    - *Offer sips of drinks as they probably won't be producing much saliva.*

- *Encourage. Eating can become less pleasurable and hard work. Don't immediately accept if they indicate they don't want any more. It may just be that they need a break.*
    - *Have a break.*
    - *Warm it up again.*
    - *Have some yourself (on a separate plate, obviously!).*
    - *Put it on a new plate so it looks appetising again.*
    - *Offer something different.*

Dysphagia in Layman's Terms

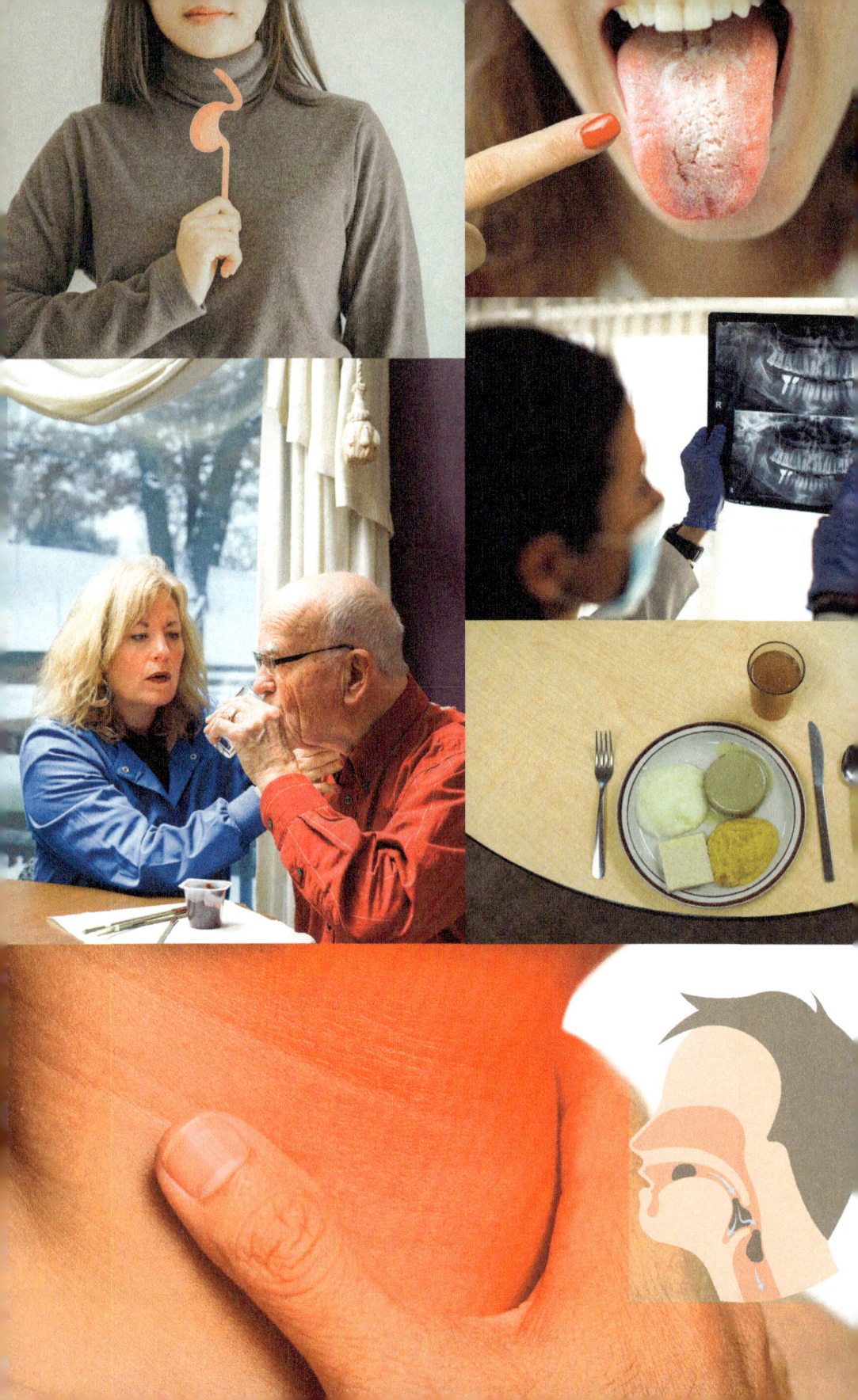

Dysphagia in Layman's Terms

To be honest, I'd never heard of Dysphagia until after my father had died. Even then, I thought it was something that only happened 'right at the end' to 'some people' who have Parkinson's Disease, Motor Neurone Disease or after a stroke.

Oh no… over the past few years, I've learnt it is so much more common (and therefore a bigger problem) than that. In fact dysphagia affects around 11% of adults living in the community, in the UK (Holland et al, 2011). This rises to up to 27% of older adults living at home in 2016 (Madhavan et al, 2016).

Dysphagia is just the medical (Greek and Latin derived) name for "swallowing difficulties".

Swallowing is actually a really complicated process where lots of things can go wrong. 50 pairs of muscles and many nerves are employed to get food from the mouth to the stomach. This happens in three stages.

1. Firstly, obviously, we have to chew our food so it is the right size, shape and consistency to travel. It comes in a variety of textures and sizes but has to hit the back of the throat in a fairly uniform puree. So the tongue moves the food around and around, mixing it with any saliva produced and taking it to the teeth to crush. During this stage, the back of the mouth is tightly shut by muscles to prevent food or liquid leaking down the throat or windpipe.

Problems here will cause massive difficulties with eating. As we age, our tongue muscles often lose their tone, along with our face, jaw and throat muscles. Teeth loosen, break and can fall out or get removed. Tooth ache and ill-fitting dentures are a very common cause of dysphagia. The third problem is a lack of saliva. There are many reasons why the body produces less saliva... certain medications like diuretics, beta blockers, PPIs (acid reflux treatment) antidepressants and antihistamines can all reduce or change saliva production. Chemotherapy and radiotherapy can cause massive problems with changing the acidity of saliva and causing mouth ulcers and tooth decay. Things that can help are sometimes quite simple:

    a. Seeing a dentist, if that is at all possible. The mere act of getting to the dentist's chair can be a feat in itself sometimes with accessibility issues, however.
    b. Checking that someone is still able to brush all their teeth. Stiff shoulders and hands may mean oral hygiene has gone a little awry.
    c. There are many saliva replacements to buy at pharmacies or online.
    d. Speech and Language Therapists, Physiotherapists and Occupational Therapists can give advice on exercises for facial muscle strength.
    e. If all else fails, you can get ready meals that are already finely chopped or pureed. They don't taste as bad as they sound!

2. Secondly, when the tongue has pushed the food to the back of the mouth, where the pharynx is, the muscles should automatically swallow. The larynx (voicebox) should close tightly and breathing automatically stops, in order to prevent food or liquid entering our lungs.

This is when aspiration is most likely to happen. Aspiration is when food or liquid leaks into the lungs. This causes coughing and pain initially. However, it is quite possibly the most worrying consequence of dysphagia. The food or drink can cause long term damage and scarring on the lungs, but also cause aspiration pneumonia. Basically, the foreign bodies can be a seat of infection that is virtually impossible to treat as the food has nowhere to go. This can be caused by slow, longer term damage due to tiny amounts of liquid leaking into the lungs over a period of time, or by a single event. This is why pneumonia is often stated on a death certificate.

Problems with swallowing are usually caused by muscle weakness, or tightening, due to aging or certain nerve and muscle disorders. If you have muscle tightening due to certain neurological or muscular conditions, Botox can help, as can other muscle relaxants.

Ways to try to prevent aspiration:

a. As we've always been told… sit as upright as we can. Having an upright posture increases tongue pressure to help with the swallow. Anyone lying in bed to eat should have their back supported to enable sitting up. It is best to stay sitting up for up to an hour after a meal too. Leaning forward or being 'hunched over' is just as hindering for a good swallow, so encourage a straight back.
b. If you think there might be an issue with leaky aspiration, then give thickened drinks, soups, jellies and milkshakes for fluid intake. Thin watery drinks tend to get into the lungs more easily.

c. Don't encourage conversation at mealtimes or interesting TV programmes. "Don't talk with your mouth full" has full medical backing! A bit of classical music in the background often keeps people focussed on eating.

3. Thirdly, we have the bit where the food is pushed down the oesophagus into the stomach. This usually takes about 3 seconds, however, this can slow down as we get older and our muscles weaken and / or stiffen. If, when you eat, you feel like something is getting stuck in your throat, or have an uncomfortable feeling behind the breastbone during or after eating, you probably have a problem with the oesophagus.

There are a few reasons why you may get pain or discomfort, here, while eating. The most common is a history of acid reflux (or GERD: Gastroesophageal Reflux Disease). If acid has been flowing back up from the stomach, it will have damaged the lining of the oesophagus, causing ulcers or scar tissue. This then narrows the oesophagus causing food to back up, resulting in vomiting. Barrett's Oesophagus is another problem where the leaked stomach acid makes the lining of the oesophagus change, to resemble the lining of the small intestine. This can have no symptoms but increases your risk of cancer in the area.

The only ways to help with reflux and pain are:
   a. Sitting up while and after eating, using gravity to help the food go downwards into the stomach.
   b. The best way to keep acid reflux down is to take Protein Pump Inhibitors (PPIs) but these are not meant to be taken for more than 8 weeks at a time (And they reduce your production of saliva). If they don't work, you may be offered an H2 Receptor Antagonist, such as Famotidine.

  c. Don't eat within 3 – 4 hours of bed time if possible.
  d. Don't wear tight fitting clothes around the waist.
  e. Smoking and drinking alcohol are best avoided.
  f. Do eat small portions and chew well.
  g. Take an over the counter antacid before each meal.

For all of the above, a visit to the GP is, without doubt, advised. GPs can refer you to Speech and Language Therapists, Occupational Therapists and Physiotherapists. They will also refer you to ENT specialists, if investigations are necessary.

Final Words

Thank you for reading my book. When I was caring for my father, I found there was so little information about how to deal with his loss of appetite. I just wanted someone to tell me how to encourage him to eat more, and what it was that he should actually be eating.

I cannot stress highly enough how important good nutrition is to our quality of life as we age. I have learnt so much in the last 6 years and I wanted to share it with you.

If we can increase the nutrition of the aging population, we can keep them stronger. If we do this, we should be able to lower hospital admissions and shorten the length of stays. This will release much needed beds for the acutely unwell and for people needing treatment.

The NHS wasn't designed to keep the frail and elderly on their wards, long term. However, sadly, cottage hospitals and recuperation centres have been closed, just as the population is living longer. Now, care and nursing homes are understaffed and many have closed in the last few years. We are looking after our elderly relatives much more at home, these days, and, as with parenting, it doesn't come with a manual!

I don't make any claims that my guidance will stop anyone from falling off the cliff at the end of life… but keeping our loved ones stronger for longer is so important. You just cannot beat good nutrition and gentle exercise.

Mary Merheim

Appendix Sample Week Menu

	Monday	Tuesday	Wednesday	Thursday	Friday	Saturday	Sunday
Breakfast	Greek full fat yoghurt with fruit and ginger	Fortified Scrambled eggs with spinach	Overnight oats with banana and frozen strawberries,	Smashed avocado and salmon	Banana pancake Fruit, honey	Porridge with cream, nuts and cinnamon	Peanut butter and banana on toast
Snack	Cheesy courgette muffin	Apple slices and cheese	Pate on toast	Melon and mixed nuts	Egg sandwich squares	Pear slices and chocolate dip	Hummus, crackers and grapes
Lunch	Quiche and mixed vegetables	Fishcakes and avocado with herb mayo	Tinned sardines and cream cheese on toast	Mushroom and cheese omelette	Chicken and vegetable soup with cheese	Baked sweet potato, cheese and baked beans	Roast chicken, mash, peas, carrots
Snack	Mixed nuts and dark chocolate	Peanut butter brownie	Apple crumble bites	Wholemeal scone with cream and jam	Blueberry muffin	Carrot cake slice	Crumble and nut ice cream
Dinner	Salmon with sweet potato mash, wilted spinach and watercress	Chicken stir fry with nut butter, mushrooms, green beans	Beef and vegetable chilli with rice and soured cream	Lentil cottage pie with broccoli and peas	Fish and chips mushy peas	Baked eggs with mackerel and spinach	Scotch egg, cheese and mixed bean salad
Dessert	Banana custard	Chocolate and avocado mousse	Jelly and fruit with ice cream	Nut ice cream sundae with fruit and chocolate sauce	Tinned peaches and custard	Apple puree and cream	Rice pudding and fruit puree

Resources and References

Contacts/Websites

IDDSI
The International Dysphagia Diet Standardisation Initiative that offers guidelines and support for swallowing problems. htttps://iddsi.org/

Dementia UK
https://www.dementiauk.org

Age UK
https://www.ageuk.org.uk

British Nutrition Foundation
https://www.nutrition.org.uk/life-stages/older-people/

References

Good Nutrition:

1. https://agsjournals.onlinelibrary.wiley.com/doi/full/10.1111/jgs.15592
2. https://www.sheffield.ac.uk/healthy-lifespan/news/more-half-older-people-dont-consume-enough-protein-stay-healthy
3. www.ncbi.nlm.nih.gov/pmc/articles/PMC3607063/
4. https://www.ncbi.nlm.nih.gov/pmc/articles/PMC6117694/
5. https://www.ncbi.nlm.nih.gov/pmc/articles/PMC3402070/
6. https://www.ncbi.nlm.nih.gov/pubmed/21897776
7. www.lifehack.org/605575/fish-oil-supplements-to-boost-memory
8. https://pubmed.ncbi.nlm.nih.gov/25592004/
9. https://www.medicalnewstoday.com/articles/300219
10. (https://www.ncbi.nlm.nih.gov/pmc/articles/PMC8463376/)
11. (CJ bates et al, 'Micronutrients: highlights and research challenges

from the 1994–5 National Diet and Nutrition Survey of people aged 65 years and over' British Journal of Nutrition (1999), 82, 7–15)
12. https://www.ncbi.nlm.nih.gov/pmc/articles/PMC9967583/
13. https://pubmed.ncbi.nlm.nih.gov/32810309/
14. https://www.ncbi.nlm.nih.gov/pmc/articles/PMC6690912/

Simple 'Hacks' to Increase Good Nutrition:

15. Mozaffarian D. Dairy Foods, Obesity, and Metabolic Health: The Role of the Food Matrix Compared with Single Nutrients. Adv Nutr. 2019;10(5):917S-923S. doi:10.1093/advances/nmz053
16. Drouin-chartier JP, Côté JA, Labonté MÈ, et al. Comprehensive Review of the Impact of Dairy Foods and Dairy Fat on Cardiometabolic Risk. Adv Nutr. 2016;7(6):1041-1051. doi:10.3945/an.115.011619
17. https://www.verywellfit.com/how-full-fat-dairy-keeps-you-lean-4158951
18. https://www.wsh.nhs.uk/CMS-Documents/Patient-leaflets/NutritionandDieteticService/6375-1-High-calorific-snacks-sheet.pdf

Hydration:

19. https://pubmed.ncbi.nlm.nih.gov/21450118/

Dysphagia in Layman's Terms:

Holland et al 2011:
https://www.practicenursing.com/content/clinical/dysphagia-in-the-older-person-an-update/#B19

Madhavan et al, 2016:
https://www.practicenursing.com/content/clinical/dysphagia-in-the-older-person-an-update/#B26

About the Author

Mary Merheim's father lost his appetite in later years, so she started looking for solutions and things that would tempt him to eat.

As well as currently being a Nutrition Advisor to the Elderly, a Dementia Activities Coordinator in a Care Home, and an End of Life Doula, Mary is also the founder and CEO of Grandbar Snacks Ltd, who make cakes packed with good calories.

Mary lives in rural Gloucestershire with her two dogs: Bean and Sprout!

Printed in Great Britain
by Amazon